IN SEARCH OF
FREEZER MEAT

*A Story of the Male Mental Health Crisis
Caused by Erectile Dysfunction and the Only
True Cure No One is Talking About...a Penis Implant*

Sharay "Punisher" Hayes

First printing May 2025
ISBN: 979-8-9987806-0-8
Library of Congress Control Number: 2025909037

The information provided in this book is for general informational purposes only and is not intended as, nor should it be considered a substitute for, professional medical advice, diagnosis, or treatment. Always seek the advice of your physician or other qualified health provider with any questions you may have regarding a medical condition, treatment, or health concern.

Never disregard professional medical advice or delay in seeking it because of something you have read in this book. The author and publisher are not medical professionals and do not claim to diagnose, treat, or cure any medical conditions. Reliance on any information provided in this book is solely at your own risk.

The author and publisher disclaim any liability for any adverse effects that may result from the use or application of the information contained herein.

ACKNOWLEDGMENTS

I would like to thank my dad for his support and inspiration! He's always been my biggest fan, and anything I attempt to do, he believes in and supports me fully. Our friendship over the last few years has been one of the brightest spots in my life, and I'm ecstatic that your joy and enjoyment of life were the biggest motivations for writing this book. I love you, dude!

To Brittany: You were my first friend who took the time to read my story when it was, honestly, a complete mess. Opening your home over the Xmas holiday to use as a writer's retreat, and immersing yourself as a lesbian woman in a book about dicks, was the best experience I've had with you in our 15-plus-year friendship. Your feedback, encouragement, belief in what I was doing, and hysterical laughter at my stories were truly the fuel I needed to get this done. Your stamp of approval made me believe, and I will always be grateful for you and your help.

To Thomas, Augustine, and Andre, three of my oldest and closest friends: Getting someone to take the time to read your book is not easy. Life be life'n, but you found the time and gave me the boosts to keep going, and I definitely needed it. Sincerely, thank you.

To Adam, Kofi, and Kevin Words: Thanks for tolerating me and my crazy stories during our group phone conversations. We would jump on the line to talk sports, and eventually I would hijack the moment with some crazy story. Your collective positive responses, enjoyment, laughter, and occasional "Dude, you need to write a fucking book," is where this all started. Thank you for accepting me as me, and for your nonjudgmental support of my truths—no matter how crazy they were—which made me comfortable enough to share them with everyone.

To Deonne, Jessica, and Tango—my visionary team that helped bring my project to life: Your patience, guidance, and wisdom were everything. The Doctors to my Frankenstein!

To Ahmed, Jude, Armondo, Fran, Jeff, Dino, Sherraine, Chanell, Shar, Ten, Matt, Drae, Ashley, Ladawn, Betty, Tamika H, Stharling, Jay, and Perfect: I just want to thank you all for the roles you played in my life. When everything was quietly crumbling, you guys were the glue that held me together... and the most beautiful part is, you didn't even know it. ♥

Lastly, to anyone who has touched my life in any way: Thank you as well, because all my experiences ultimately led me here... and I am proud and grateful for it.

So, First Thing's First to Keep My Lawyer Happy

Please take note: I am NOT a doctor, and what I'm sharing in this book is not medical advice—it's a compilation of everything I've learned about penis problems and solutions based on my line of work and my personal experience fixing my own issues. The first thing I always tell guys that come to me for advice is this—before you do anything, try anything, or take anything, go to your doctor first, because you need to rule out physical issues before you address the rest. Nine times out of 10, their physical health is fine, but there are certain important factors that only a doctor can diagnose. Doctors can tell you directly the best way to solve your issue, so it's always worth it to get things checked out. We men tend to think "Hey, I'll just deal with it" and adjust. But look at your sexual health like sitting in your living room and it's on fire... do you just say, "I'll deal with it and adjust" or do you spring into action and stop the fire? Of course, you do everything you can to put that fire out. So see a doctor if you can. Knowing what's up down there helps big time with your ability to do something proactive about it.

TABLE OF CONTENTS

From the Author

When you hear the term "erectile dysfunction," you almost always think of a physical problem. Truth is, it's a much, much bigger mental problem. In this book, I want to share how the mental issue played a part in my being a shell of myself as a man—how it lowers your standards, your self-esteem, and your drive, plus affects the focus you would normally put into other aspects of life. Being consumed with focusing on your sexual issues brings on depression, hurts relationships, changes the whole dynamic of relationships, and wreaks havoc on a man's life in so many ways.

I will talk about how it's being ignored, how it's not being put at the forefront for men to really seek help past the physical fix of trying to get their erection back. I don't want you to feel like you're on an island alone to suffer the consequences like I once was. Whatever may be the remedy for you, I want to encourage men to seek this out. Ultimately, I believe the only true fix is an implant. But no one is talking about it. It's not just an option for eighty-year-old men who have had prostate surgery. It is something men should be more proactive about and looking to get—if you have the means—because it actually gives you a reset. It gives you the possibility to reset all the mental issues that erectile dysfunction can create. It is a mental health crisis. If you know…you know.

PREFACE

My Dad, My Dude, My Ultimate Inspiration

This book is about how I faced my fears and fixed my erectile dysfunction—and completely changed my life for the (MUCH) better. But before I get into the details of my journey, from growing up in Harlem to becoming a wildly successful male stripper to getting a life-changing penis implant, I've got to tell you about my dad.

My dad is a 67-year-old disabled veteran and a very cool dude. Everybody loves the guy. He's hilariously funny, super social, and talks to everybody. He was the gangster guy in the 'hood, did some time in jail when he was younger—got out, got back with my mom, and turned his life around.

When my mom passed away in 2004, Dad was still a fairly young guy and still quite good-looking. Of course, there would be some time mourning and getting over Mom, but at some point, I realized that he never really picked up his life again in terms of dating and socializing. A few years after my mom died, he dated one woman for a long period of time. Then he traveled and met a woman here and there, but over the many years since my mother's passing, there had been very little noticeable romantic activity.

Dad retired, moved to South Carolina, and bought his dream house. He was living his life and was set up pretty nicely with what we guys believe are chick magnets—he had the drop-top Mercedes SL and the Cadillac Escalade—fit, funny, and well-financed.

When I would visit him, I'd see he had all his boxes checked, but he still seemed like a loner, and I was asking myself, "What's going on?"

A few years ago, when I said, "Dad, I'm thinking about getting a penis implant," his reaction was, "What? No freaking way. Why would you do something like that, Man? You are absolutely crazy. You don't need to do nothing like that."

This is actually the normal reaction when you tell someone you want an implant and trust me, I've heard this a lot, and we'll get into that later in the book.

Come to find out, my dad had been getting his own prescriptions from the VA: Viagra, Cialis, and dick injections, but he wasn't using any of it. Dad is a hustle man and doesn't say no to anything free, so he's going to get every prescription or whatever they offer, whether he needs it or not. So he had all these ED meds sitting in the drawer, and they're not being used, so he started giving them to me. He told me he was good to go and didn't need to take it, which was super impressive to me and damaging at the same time.

I said to myself, "If he's in his sixties and didn't need it, what the fuck is wrong with me?"

But with his encouragement, I started using the medication, and lo and behold, I still got the implant (I'll write more about why that often happens later).

After I got my implant, I was fucking overjoyed, and I told my dad about how I was having some of the best sex of my life. I explained how my implant worked better than my original penis at its peak and candidly shared all the fun I was having.

So finally, Dad, who, mind you, was completely against the idea of me getting an implant, said, "Man, what's that doctor's number? I'm doing that shit."

Sure enough, Dad was having erectile issues, too. For exactly how long and how severe we didn't get into, but that was my first indication that something was going on with him. So, I walked him through the process, told him how to contact the doctor, and what he needed to do in terms of getting it covered by his insurance. And a calendar year almost to the day I got mine done, my dad got approved and had his surgery.

After Dad healed and put his new power tool to work for the first time, he literally called me and thanked me every day for the next six months.

"Thank you, thank you, thank you! It changed my life. You saved my life. I wake up every day with my sore back, hurting knees, and old man pain, but still with the biggest smile on my face I've ever had. You don't understand; my life is renewed, I feel reborn, and I'm so happy."

Now, all of a sudden, that loner guy who was parked in the house binging Netflix series is all over town. And he's got more girls than me, and—even more impressive—they're all younger than me!

Dad has been on a roll!

"What the fuck are you taking?" was the question my father's lady friend, who was forty-one years old, recently asked him when he was instantly ready for another round of sex.

Playing stupid, he responded, "What do you mean, taking something? I have no idea what you're talking about." They had already been going at it all day long.

"They just can't get enough of me," he giddily told me on one of our daily calls as he recapped his sexcapades like an episode of *SportsCenter*.

He'd be at the barbershop with his old buddies, talking shit about how he took a part-time job as a plumber 'cause a bunch of pipe needed to be laid around town.

A side effect of having an implant is your dick is significantly bigger when soft than a normal penis, so you walk around with a serious bulge. Boy, does he love this! Now I've got my dad sending me Amazon links of gray sweatpants he's ordering to put his piece on proper display.

"The dick print gets them every time," he says.

It got to the point where he actually started complaining, as he would call me whispering, "I can't get this damn girl outta here." Another early forties babe came by on a Wednesday to stay with him for the Labor Day weekend. He said she was supposed to leave on Sunday, but he couldn't get her to leave. She stayed until the next Wednesday.

Halfway through her stay, she asked him, "What the fuck is going on?"

Dad had been Rodney-King beating (sexually) her all day long. She insisted he tell her what was going on.

"This shit is not normal," she said. "What the fuck is happening?"

There is truly no way for a woman to tell you have an implant.

Dad laughed and finally gave in and said, "Listen, I got an implant. I can do this all day," in his Captain America voice.

Her response? "Hey, look, the women your age can't appreciate this, but I can! I'm going to have a ball."

He said for the rest of the trip, she must've showered four times a day. Every time she came out of the shower, she grabbed his balls and said, "Let's go."

They just cracked up about it, which was a relief for my dad, as you never know how someone will react to an implant, but they had straight fun with it. Which, believe it or not, is the norm.

Most women, when they hear you have an implant, become intrigued. I mean, it does make sense. Why wouldn't a woman be excited about a man she's into having a never-ending erection? Since Dad got the implant, he's been an Energizer Bunny to the nth degree. And this is going to sound weird, but I've never been so happy for another man to use his dick. I'm more invested in my dad's sex life than my own. But most importantly, my dad is a completely new man. I don't even know this guy. When I saw the joy in my dad's reincarnation—the glow, the energy, the lust for life, the happiness—all the things that came with him just being able to feel like a man again—it once again reaffirmed my own decision to change my life with an implant. Because everything my dad was feeling was the same thing I was feeling. It saved his life, and it saved mine, too! Seeing the way my dad's life changed made it clear—I needed to write this book.

It's a no-brainer. There are a lot of men who could use this boost, and no one's talking about it. We need to be talking about it because of all the men out there who think their lives are over—that they've peaked sexually and it's all downhill from there. I was one of them…so was my dad. But we chose not to give up on our dicks. We wanted to be not just capable of sex in some watered-down shell of our self-version, we wanted to be the men we were confident and proud of being sexually—something all men should never give up on. Seeing my dad return to prominence in his sexuality was all I needed to see to try and motivate others the way I did for him.

So my inspiration is my dad, Al Hayes, aka DDP: Daddy Dick Print.

INTRODUCTION

Our Cocks, Ourselves: Why Do Dicks Loom So Large in Our Imaginations?

Can you imagine having the best sex of your life at 50? My name is Sharay Punisher Hayes, and I certainly have been. I've reached my sex pinnacle way later than one would expect, and it's not because of some super gorgeous women I'm hooking up with, or some type of fantasy sexual lifestyle I stumbled upon. It's very simple... my dick finally works right! Nah, fuck that, that's an understatement. It's more like at 50 years old, my dick works better than it ever has in my entire life by far.

Like, imagine if you had some X-Men mutant superpower where you could time travel and replace your current dick with a dick from your past self. But your current dick is still the greatest of all your past dicks? Better than your 1992 season or 1993, and even 1996 when you won the slinging dick championship, scoring title, plus league MVP. Imagine if Michael Jordan, in the final year of his NBA career at 40 years old, suddenly had the same athleticism as his 22-year-old self but added never-ending stamina to the equation! This would obviously be an unheard-of possibility to achieve. But this is exactly the position my dick is in right now—all the knowledge, smarts, and wisdom combined with elite physical ability and stamina. How did I achieve these miraculous feats? I, at 47 years old, got a penis implant!

1

Now I know what you are thinking. "Penis implant? Fuck no. This guy's crazy!" And I don't blame you. When I first heard of it, I had the same reaction. I actually thought it was the funniest shit I'd ever heard. I learned through a mutual friend that a buddy of mine had an implant, and I instantly became the Dave Chappelle of implant jokes: "You and your Reebok pump dick." "Dude got the Inspector Gadget dick." "Go-go gadget dick!" I mean, I couldn't stop telling jokes. I thought it was hilarious until... my dick stopped working. And boy was that humble pie served when the same guy, who I clowned behind his back, I was calling every other day, gratefully trying to get any information he was willing to share. Luckily for me, he was cool as hell and helped me in any way he could in the process of getting my implant, and let me tell you, that was tremendously needed. For this to be such an effective cure for ED, it's an option never talked about. So now, I guess it's my turn to pay it forward. Help my fellow bros struggling through a non-cooperative dick.

But I'm going to take it a step further because getting my implant didn't just correct my ability to get an erection. It ended a 20-year journey of struggling with onset ED that, to be honest with you, I had no idea I was struggling with at all. Not only did the onset of ED affect the obvious, which was my boner, but the deteriorating process over two decades had crept into every aspect of my life. It went from a physical issue to a mental health problem that affected me, my partners, my friends, and my life as a whole negatively—a negative effect I was completely blinded to until after my implant. But you don't see the chaos when you are in the eye of the storm. When you come out on the other side, you clearly see the path of destruction.

So many men are blind to the toll this process is taking on our lives. As men, we kind of operate from a mindset of "it is what it is," and whatever struggles we go through, if we don't have the answer, then we just find a way to accept it. Just live with it. I'm here to tell you that's not the way. But I'm not a doctor or a medical professional on any level. I'm just a guy who couldn't live with "it is what it is" as a mindset for my worsening erectile dysfunction. I literally tried every motherfucking thing under the sun to fix my dick. My dick not working was not an option, and now I want to share with you my extensive knowledge and journey to the promised land of dick rejuvenation. Welcome to the *Cockbook*—learn what to do when your dick lets you down!

Why did I write this book? Very easy answer. Over the last 5 years before my implant, I really hit a place of desperation and frantically wanted to correct my ED issues. Now let me be clear: my dick still worked, and when it did, it was fantastic. But let me tell you, he was one unreliable motherfucker! I never knew if he was going to show up for work (get hard) or decide to go home mid-shift (go soft in the act). And the worst part was he refused to go to work if he had to wear office attire (condoms). Like, this dude was just the worst. So, this toxic unreliable relationship with my dick compelled me to seek answers.

I ended up buying tons of books and reading countless articles, but what I noticed was none of the info I found was personable or truly helpful. Just some medical ED info with the typical cause, effect, possible solution mumbo jumbo. Info that I guess made sense, but nothing I could relate to. So, then I found myself on forums where guys did post some good info from time to time, but for every interesting helpful forum thread I read, there were 20 that were just a waste of time, so this process was tedious and extremely time-consuming.

Then I decided to seek advice from my circle of friends by being candidly open about my struggles on an uncomfortable crackhead level: "I'll suck yo dick for some ED help." No seriously, a convo with me was like:

"Hey, Ray, you see the game last night?"

"Nah, bro, was too busy trying to figure out my ED problem, my dick tripping—speaking of tripping dicks, you got any Viagra?"

The awkwardness would crash in like a tidal wave, but I didn't give a fuck. Crackheads need crack, and stud muffins need a working dick! So fuck the awkwardness, I just kept talking. Ironically, what would happen is almost every guy I blindsided with the ED convo would get comfortable with my very open sharing of my struggles and start to spill their guts with tales of their own problems. "Shit, we all fucked up out here!"

Being a highly sought-after male stripper with all these women after me was a dream stud scenario for almost all my buddies, so when the conversations started, they were shocked to hear that even in my position of so-called 'sexual prosperity', I was struggling just like they were.

A non-cooperative penis can mess with any guy, no matter how great the circumstances may seem to their friends! Most of us hide our life struggles, especially when we are pedestaled by our peers. But I've always preferred to be a straight shooter and very open with my personal issues, so this has created a space where guys become very comfortable sharing their own struggles openly with me.

So, obviously, when "Mr. Dream Stud" spoke of ED struggles, it instantly placed me as the ED specialist. Instead of getting help from my friends, I began being the go-to guy in my circle for remedies. I would do tons of research and share the info with my buddies, or whoever was comfortable enough to have the convo with me. I was a real-life version of Will Smith's character Hitch, but only for dicks (that sounded all fucked up, but it's true).

As time went on, it became clear that what was needed to help me navigate this difficult journey was the voice of a guy who was going through the same shit as me, giving me the playbook and coaching me through this tough game of ED, making it normal and okay to be dealing with this, letting me know I wasn't alone with this problem and, most importantly, to not give up on finding a solution—NO MATTER WHAT! But that wasn't available for me.

So here I am trying to be that guy for you. This book is a conversation between two homies who have been struggling with our dicks, and I'm just trying to share everything to do and not to do to get your shit back to where it needs to be. It's crucial to address this issue! It's much deeper and more impactful than just your physical ability. It's about your mental health, masculinity, and ability to truly be fulfilled in life, all of which are being negatively affected that you may not be seeing at the moment. And if worse comes to worst, at least you learn how to be the prime Michael Jordan of your dick life at 50! I'd say it's a win-win.

So, if you're still reading at this point, I'm going to assume you are on board with the idea of us as two homies having the conversation of "What the fuck is going on with my dick?" Chances are, if you're ready to have it with me, you've been having it with yourself for quite some time already. Maybe you're thinking about whether your dick is "normal." Maybe you're worried about whether it's functioning correctly or pleasing your partner the right way. Maybe you're obsessed about whether it's big enough. Maybe you have my issue, and you are obsessively worrying about getting it up when it's called to duty. Maybe it's a whole bunch of other wild things only you and your brain will ever know about. But one thing is clear: you know you need to do something about it.

I'm guessing you have already spent endless hours scouring Internet message boards and watching YouTube videos about dick problems and solutions. Tried the typical Viagra/Cialis, but you know something is still off. If you are like me (I really hope not), you also ordered about 30 bottles of different types of snake oil products with names like "Bone-Atron," the new wonder erection/testosterone booster. Possibly passed by the anti-aging clinic for five rounds of the latest Frankenstein electric shock dick wave treatment quackery that is said to enhance blood flow strong enough to revive a corpse (I really did this, smh). Or you're even worse—like many of us—you have just accepted your fate of a poorly functioning penis, blamed it on Father Time or some other issue, and made peace with the inability to use your piece. This is the madness we go through over our dicks, and I'm here to tell you, my guy, it's way too common these days. A lot of your buddies are doing the same shit and just keeping it quiet. I believe the silence around the issue just sets us up to be taken advantage of by these false hope remedies.

But before we dive into the solution, let's first truly take a look at the possible problems, and for most of us, they started years before our dick started acting up. Shit, in my case, it started before I even had sex.

The Sad Story of Wack-Dick Will

When I was at Junior High School 43 in Harlem, at the ripe old age of 14, I lost my virginity, but not before the terrifying story of "Wack-Dick Will," my best friend in school. We attended an inner-city (aka hood) junior high school in Harlem that, for some odd reason, went from 7th to 9th grade. So finally making it to senior year, we were now officially the cool kids in school. Now, of course, being the cool kid in a hood junior high school in 1988 had one of two very specific requirements: you had to either be really tough, as in bordering on juvenile delinquent, which we were certainly not, or you had to be "the man" with the ladies and smashing buns on a high frequency, which we were not either. But oh boy, were we good at lying about it. The truth is, we were both still virgins, but the word on the street would have you believe we were the inspiration for Bang Bros, the porn company. Our fake sex stories, which started in 7th grade, were so solid, straight-faced, and unwavering by senior year that I'm sure we both would have passed lie detector tests and intense interrogations by the CIA. There was no doubt in anyone's mind in our school that we were experienced lovers, and it was a cool rep to have.

Finally, for Will, the years of lying miraculously paid off as his constant bragging about his abilities piqued the interest of one of the little hot-in-the-pants girls named Sue, who just couldn't resist the opportunity to see these amazing skills Will had. So one day during the after-school program, Sue took Will into the staircase for some action while a few of us waited in the hallway. Now, I can remember this like it happened yesterday because it will be imprinted in my mind for the rest of time. Will was the first to walk out of the staircase, and when I tell you... it was my first time seeing true joy and elation. The smile on his face was wide and infectious. His face was glowing, just radiating happiness. It was clear this was the best moment of his young life, and I was truly moved to happiness for him as if I had just gotten some buns. Will walked over and gave me a high five with the exuberance of someone who hit the game-winning, buzzer-beater shot for the championship!

About seven seconds later, Sue emerged from the staircase with a look on her face that I could only describe as fitting for someone who just stepped in diarrhea in a dirty gas station bathroom... barefoot. The look of disgust was compounded by her yelling to whoever could hear, "THIS MOTHERFUCKER WAS TRASH! HE LASTED FUCKING TWO MINUTES—OMG, IT WAS SO WACK!" She just went on and on about his poor performance and, honestly speaking, Will really didn't have much of a defense because it did appear they were in and out of the staircase in under 90 seconds. So her actually calling him a two-minute brother was stat-padding him by about 30 seconds.

Will's joyous expression quickly changed as if the referees reviewed his game-winning shot and waived it off because he released it after time expired. By the next day, everyone in school knew of Will's epic fail. No one could stop talking about it. His cool guy reputation and senior life were pretty much ruined! Thus, the nickname Wack-Dick Will was born, and followed him until we graduated. It was so cemented to him that it became casual convo. For example, if someone said, "I hung out with Will yesterday," a casual response would be, "Which one? Short Will or Wack Dick?" He even got a nickname for his nickname, as people who were close to him called him WDW for short. Poor Will—from stud to dud in 90 seconds.

About two months after Will's sad moment, it was finally my moment of truth. Over that time span, I got my first girlfriend, and she gave me the green light to pop her cherry. So, of course, I was psyched but nervous as hell. The closest I'd been to some actual pussy was my neighbor's cat, so I was pretty much clueless. I was 14, so I couldn't really have girls over to my place, so I ended up at my 17-year-old neighbor's house for some privacy. She came by, and it was my moment of truth, and I was failing miserably because, lo and behold, I couldn't even find the fucking hole! For about 20 minutes straight, I poked everything possible to try to gain entry, and it was just not happening. As the frustration mounted, I eventually lost my erection and gave up—it was time to leave anyway, as my boy's mom was almost home.

Sadly, I put my girl in a taxi and was immediately greeted by my boy with the "How was it?" Q and A.

At that moment, my disappointment couldn't muster another lie, so I honestly admitted, "I never got it in," in a defeated voice.

Expecting to be clowned for the failure, to my surprise, my boy just laughed and said, "Ah man, why didn't you grab the Vaseline off my dresser?"

Vaseline! Why the hell didn't I think of that?

So fast forward a week later, and my girlfriend finally gave me another shot. It was a Friday afternoon, and I managed to sneak her into my bedroom while Grandma was locked into an intense episode of *The Price is Right*. I got her in the room, shut the door, assumed our positions for sex, and guess what?

Drum roll, please...

I STILL COULDN'T FIND THE FUCKING HOLE! Another session of poke, poke, poke, poke, poke, and nothing for 20 to 25 minutes. As the frustration was mounting, yet again, and my erection was about to call it quits from discouragement, I suddenly started to hear my boy's voice quietly echoing like a ghost at a séance: "Grab the Va-se-line-line-line. The Va-se-line-line-line."

Yes! I needed Vaseline! But wait! I didn't have any! Stressed and slightly frantic, I had no choice but to use what I had. I grabbed a bottle of Jergens lotion off the dresser, squirted the equivalent of a small bowl of oatmeal worth on my junk, and went to town. That Jergens was a game changer, and as I penetrated with ease, "I'm in! I'm in!" I thought joyously, finally experiencing the elation I saw on Will's face when he walked out of the stairs. But fuck that, I was not going out like him in two minutes! No way!

Now in my mind, I was more than prepared for this moment. I had easily put in well over 1,000 hours of sex-simulated masturbation. I had beat my dick off in every position of the Kama Sutra...twice. So I was ready! But like any normal 14-year-old boy, by the third pump, it was like I was shot with a taser; my body did an intense epileptic shimmy, and of course, I came almost instantly. WHELP! As my lifeless body collapsed on top of her, cross-eyed and drooling from the best 17 seconds of my life, I immediately faced the fear of "Sheesh, if Will was clowned for being a two-minute brother, what's going to happen to me after my 20 sorry-ass seconds?"

Just being a firsthand witness to the horrible, ego-crushing story of Wack-Dick Will, I sat around the entire weekend scared to go to school worried that Janell, genuinely a very nice girl, was going to fucking ruin my entire life and tell the whole school that I was a "Two-minute Brother" (ironically, at the time, that was the name of a hit rap song clowning guys for coming too fast by a group called Bitches With Problems).

Luckily, Janell didn't say a word, and all was well with my reputation, at least. Now my mental state was another story, as from that moment on, I went into almost every sexual encounter with pressure to perform, and that's where it all started. The seeds of shame and dick doubt are planted very early in young boys. Although I avoided the embarrassment of Wack-Dick Will, I did not escape the performance anxiety and pressure of being judged as a poor lover, which, unfortunately for me, started at 14 years old. This type of mental programming happens to many of us in its own way with our early experiences, which for most of us becomes a big issue when we start to decline.

In my case, when I became a male stripper at 22, a whole extra layer of perceived potency was added to my persona.

Being a male stripper immediately attaches an expectation of your being the best lover ever. A fantasy-type experience is what most women imagine, which I wholeheartedly tried to live up to. That's when things got really complicated for me and my relationship with my dick, as my decline felt like falling off Mt. Everest.

Now, my case is extreme, but I believe we all are dealing with a form of sexual anxiety associated with early sexual pressure, living up to the hype in your prime, and sadly finding ourselves struggling to keep up with our younger selves as the decline happens.

Our Universal Dick Obsession

One of the most eye-opening things I discovered in my journey to fix my ED is that more than 50% of ED cases are all mental. Yup, absolutely nothing physically wrong with the guy. Just over time, we can develop such a fragile mental state around sex that it hampers our ability to perform. I was this same guy, and thinking back to it, I realize that this was inevitably where I would end up. Because of the sexual imprint and understanding that started at such an early age, as I was just discovering what sex was, it's called simply sexual performance anxiety. All around us is a constant message that puts pressure on your dick. I mean, sheesh— have you ever seen a movie or TV show, or listened to a couple of bars of any hip-hop song from 1980? There is a whole industry, an entire culture, and a long-ass history of men being validated by our dicks. Society keeps a clear standard in place that to be considered a high-level man, you have to be a stud sexually.

We get that message so early that I can remember lying to friends, denying I was a virgin at as young as 11 years old, making up stories of these imaginary girlfriends I had sex with to impress friends, but even worse, to avoid the shame of not being sexually active. That, at 11, is crazy.

So fast forward to adulthood, and it was still going on. On top of whatever sexual pressure you organically put on yourself, most of us still walk around standing on a tightrope of inadequacy created by the constant standard of greatness associated with being a lover. It then creeps into our inner circle, as we all have that one friend who tells these elaborate, over-the-top stories about how he banged some chick for four hours straight at her parents' house, and her mom heard the commotion and was so turned on she joined in, so he had to bang them both for another three hours. (All while you're hearing this story of a seven-hour sex session, you are hiding your intimidation because your average sex time is 8 minutes and 32 seconds.)

Or you've heard the stereotypical conversations between women swooning over sexual experiences with men who "put it down" in the bedroom, saying, "OMG, sex was so good with him! Girl, he blew my back out last night!" knowing damn well the closest you've come to blowing a back out is trying to lift two cases of water while grocery shopping. Now, most men are not directly affected by this in the moment, especially if you are functioning fine sexually, but that high standard imprinted in the back of your brain becomes a complete confidence destroyer when you start to experience the smallest struggles sexually.

Truthfully, this is a high sexual standard that very few people live by. But mentally, we are so bombarded with glorified sex tales fueled by superhuman dicks. To make matters worse, if you find yourself in a position where you believe you are not living up to the hype, the obsession just intensifies in the form of trying whatever you can to live up to it or just living silently in shame of not believing you can.

The list of these expectations goes on and on. We believe we've got to have big dicks or dicks that work at the highest level every time and all the time because we've heard it from what we believe are "trusted" sources. Basically, we've been told that if our dick isn't performing like it just won the record of the year at the Grammys, we're total motherfucking failures. This false, damaging belief is handed down from generation to generation, from fathers to sons, uncles to cousins, and neighborhood dudes on the corner who dispense advice to anyone willing to listen.

Now, this is nothing new, and the stories men absorb about their dicks are damaging and have been a crucial imprint on male sexuality for years. But I believe we have managed it pretty well up until the last 10 years. Now it's gotten tremendously worse to a toxic level. Today's message to men has created a thought process similar to what women go through about being hot from the time they're 8 until they're 90—they call that "the beauty myth." Modern women have been placed in a pressurized obsession with physical perfection that traps them in an endless spiral of hope, self-consciousness, and self-hatred as they try to fulfill society's impossible definition of "the flawless beauty." It's obvious to see how the beauty myth for women is perpetuated through countless ads for beauty enhancement over every inch of their bodies. Cosmetic surgeries for BBLs, boobs, lips, Botox, etc., are through the roof and are as common now as a yearly check-up.

This pressurized, constant attack on your self-esteem was something men were not subjected to on a daily basis through marketing platforms until now. These days, you cannot view or listen to any entertainment programming geared toward men without repeatedly seeing constant ads about Cialis, Viagra, testosterone boosters, and a host of products focused on a man's diminished sexuality. To make it worse, all the ads make reference to a woman or potential sexual partner who will benefit from your purchasing the product, indirectly putting a man's sexual performance in question. Behind the counter at the deli, gas station, or vitamin store, there's a tremendous push to enhance your dick or testosterone. It's implanting a damaging message about our sexuality that is undermining the confidence of men in the same way the beauty myth is affecting women. This message of inadequacy with our dicks is being pushed much differently than in the past, and unfortunately, it has us all sitting around googling the fuck out of what might be wrong with us all night long, but the only remedy being offered is paying money to Big Pharma or whatever zany remedy we can come up with to address the physical problem to meet a standard that should never have been forced on us in the first place. But it is what it is. This is the standard that men operate under, and more important than any pill you can take is the conversation of how this standard is messing with your mind. Because if your mind gets too far gone with these issues... there's nothing the pills can do for you. Trust me, I'm living proof of that, and I will discuss more later.

How Porn Has Warped Our Brains

Watching porn for a lot of us is also damaging in terms of the standard it imprints in a man's brain. Look, I'm a fan of porn, but the facts are the facts. Before I had sex, I based what I needed to be during sex off porn! My whole outline of sex when I got the hang of it was based on what I saw on TV. It went something like: cheesy convo with music, eat her pussy, get some head, stick it in, alternate three positions—missionary, her on top, doggie style... cum shot... the end. I practiced my strokes, rhythm, and sounds based on these three VHS tapes I found in my grandpa's room. Now, the format help was cool, which I was able to mimic pretty quickly in my sex journey, and honestly, I still use the format to this day. But the thing that was the biggest obstacle was, damn, these porn dudes' dicks are huge! There was a quiet intimidation clearly associated with what I saw on the screen and what I had in my hand. I truly felt like if life was the card game Poker, I was dealt two pair (which is okay), but these porn guys clearly all got royal flushes.

Confirmation of the Cock Illusion

I got a pervy homie named Gee who insists on videotaping himself having sex with random girls and putting it in our group chat. Just out of the blue, my phone pings, and "Oh shit, it's Gee's dick again!" Not exactly the message I want to get, but fuck it, porn is porn, so it was my duty to check it out. So the true friend I am, I watched and truly celebrated the great time my buddy was having on video. But I'm just keeping it 100... goddamn, Gee was killing me on the dick size; his shit looked fucking humongous. I was thinking to myself, *I don't want to fuck any girls after Gee, because shit might make me look bad.*

I'm not a video dude, so I clearly had never been the type to tape myself. First of all, I need tremendous focus to keep my erection up at baseline, so if I start messing with a camera while trying to fuck, I'm probably out of the game with a dick going down like a journeyman boxer vs. Mike Tyson in his prime.

So shortly after my penis implant, my boy Gee sent another one of his random hung-like-a-horse sex videos to the group chat. But now I was keeping erections; no problem. So after doing my duty of watching and admiring his work, I decided, "Hey, maybe I'll do some filming myself."

Later that night, I was hooking up with a lady friend, pulled out my camera, and got my Steven Spielberg on. A great job was done, if I say so myself, as an implant makes all things possible! Later on, when I went back to review the footage, I thought, *Holy shit, my dick looks twice the size! My shit's humongous, too. What a surprise!* The point is that a lot of this male obsession with penis size is associated with watching porn, but what is unspoken is how the camera itself, angles, and the size of the girls are a big factor in the appearance of your size. You know how they say TV puts 10 pounds on you? Well, it does wonders for your dick!

So lo and behold, all this penis pressure I had over the years from watching porn and then even more from watching Gee's videos, which was like, "Damn, this is my homie and my dick is Spud Webb to his Dikembe Mutombo!" I now realized this penis pressure was falsely imprinted. So if you've been watching porn, looking at all these big dicks, and then looking at your own dick, wondering why the world is so cruel to you, just remember, you're in the game. Just grab your camera, get the right angle, and feel better about yourself!

THE MENTAL HEALTH SPIRAL

Broken Heart Leads to Broken Cock

Like I mentioned in the earlier chapters, my sexual pressure and performance anxiety started at a young age, mainly because of a combo of porn and Wack Dick Will's story. In my teens, I was pretty sexually active and prioritized honing my skills to what I believed was a great lover for a young guy.

So when I turned 22 and decided to become a male stripper, the sexual conquest goal went bananas. It didn't help that my motivation to become a stripper was some dysfunctional heartbreak tale associated with my high school sweetheart, Tina, who I thought I was going to marry. It was a pretty serious relationship, as we were already living together in a top floor apartment at my grandparents' place. Our parents loved us together, and all in all, it seemed we were in love and perceivably very happy.

So I'm completely blindsided when, in year four of our relationship, she comes home and tells me, "I'm going to start working in a female strip club." So like any 21-year-old boyfriend in love with his girlfriend, I responded with, "No the fuck you not." Then proceeded to argue, beg, and plead for her not to, and she hit me with, "It's happening no matter what, so either you're in or out." The sucker for love I was at the time; I stayed with her and just found a way to accept it.

About a year later, she comes home and says, "I'm meeting all these men in the club, and I'm tired of being tied down, so I want to be single," and dumped me—straight cold-blooded like that. So I moved back to Harlem with my family, devastated and heartbroken, determined to get my girl back.

My master plan as a heartbroken 22-year-old—"You know what? I'm going to become a stripper, and she will see all the women after me, understand how it feels, and want me back." So I went on this determined quest to become a male stripper. After a couple of months of trying to get connected, I finally had an in. Now I just needed a stage name.

At the time, I was a pretty good basketball player and earned the nickname "The Punisher" from my West 4th Street basketball buddies, so it was simple to transition that nickname to stripping. Plus, the original name I came up with, "Caramel Mandingo," wasn't exactly ringing bells. So, Punisher it is!

Now, my plan worked to perfection because I was no more than two months into trying to be in the stripping business, and my ex-girlfriend was already intrigued and wanted to revisit our relationship! Nice! Just what I hoped for! She was very interested and wanted to see what the whole male stripping thing was about, but she wasn't ready to see me perform without knowing what to expect.

So I made a few calls and set her up to go to a show in Brooklyn that was not too far from her house. Knowing that I wasn't going to be there, I told a female friend of mine named Stacy that my ex-girl, Tina, was going to be there and to look out for her.

Small world it was, as about 10:00 a.m., the morning after the show, I got a call from Stacy, and she said, "I'm sorry, Sharay, but I have some bad news. Your ex-girl you told me about went home with one of the strippers. He's friends with my boyfriend. She's at his house now."

My heart dropped to my stomach. The pain made me numb. I was in disbelief and just wanted answers, but this was 1995, and cellphones weren't any and everywhere yet.

Finally, sometime in the afternoon, I caught my ex at home on the phone, and not only did she confirm she went home with him and fucked him, she proceeded to tell me, "You're full of shit. You not a stripper. The guy I was with is a big-time stripper, and he never heard of you." Which was true.

At that moment, I was a nobody—just a guy trying to be a stripper by showing up to places and basically begging for a chance. It was obvious she didn't give a shit about me or my feelings, and I'm crushed. My plan not only didn't get my girlfriend back, it also ushered her straight to the next man's bed. And I'm devastated.

Now, fast forward to the very next weekend, and I showed up at a male revue show in the Bronx doing the usual—making my rounds, begging for a chance to perform. I entered the dressing room and, so badly wanting to be one of the guys, I decided to introduce myself.

The first guy I walked up to, I said, "Hey, bro, I'm Punisher. Nice to meet you."

His response: "Oooo, shit, you're Punisher? Tina's man? Yooo, she got some nice fucking titties." Then he and his buddy, who was actually Stacy's boyfriend, started hysterically laughing like the audience at a Def Comedy Jam show. They were hugging each other and falling over on the couch.

It was a horrible moment for me as a young man, but I played it cool and didn't react. In this embarrassing, awkward, disrespectful moment, all I could respond with was, "Yup! You right! She do got some nice titties," and tried my best to laugh with them instead of being laughed at.

That moment changed me. I no longer believed in love, relationships, or the idea of any chance of vulnerability. I became a monster, and to me, all women were good for was sex, and they would be discarded. My heartbroken state just drove me in a way that I was going to vindicate this moment, and the first place I started was Stacy.

She wasn't dating the guy who clowned me, talking about my ex-girlfriend's titties, but she was dating his friend— Mr. Def Comedy Jam, who laughed at me. So, as they say, "revenge is a dish best served cold," and I was cold fucking the shit out of Stacy by the end of the week.

These newfound antics escalated to a decade of disconnected conquests with women. Everything sexual was a physical transaction and nothing more. What looked like a nice guy on the outside was a broken, heartless young man who knew nothing of intimacy and wanted no parts of it— only sex and fucking.

Now, I share this terrible tale to point out that a lot of men with psychogenic ED have a similar history—heartbreak and a misguided view on sex and love that created a jaded perspective that only allows you to look at sex through a very physical, superficial lens.

Over time, this disconnected place becomes numb to the response. You end up desensitized physically, and if you don't heal your heart to truly connect emotionally, your dick is going to struggle. The heartbreak was what set me down this path.

It's not a coincidence that guys who are struggling with ED can usually achieve erections with partners they have intimate bonds with and struggle with superficial, primarily physical sex. When you're young and in your prime, it doesn't matter if sex is just physical, but when you're older, make sure you are capable of connecting on all levels.

You may just discover your dick is physically fine. Your inability to look at sex on a deeper level because of past pain and trauma could be the culprit. To put it in simpler terms: it's a completely different mindset from sex with a one-night stand and sex with someone you love. Make sure you are not treating both situations with the same energy.

Every guy I've spoken to has a deep-rooted tale of heartbreak that, for a time, has hampered their ability to connect, bond, and love fully. The ones that allowed themselves to truly heal have been able to move forward and build healthy relationships.

Guys like me who couldn't let it go and carried the dysfunction over years and years, trying to keep my sexual function based on a disconnected sexual desire, are the vast majority that struggle. Our minds are detrimental to our sexual health and carrying these issues with you can derail your whole life.

The True Way We See Our Value as MEN

From age 22 to 32, I honestly will say I was living the life. These years, for men, genuinely represent your sexual peak, and your dick is a force to be reckoned with. Erections are genuinely not a problem, and sexual confidence is usually at its all-time high.

The issue here for most of us is this is where you can set your mark—meaning, how high you set your sexual bar is the place you fall from when you decline. So if you go about sex like a high-performance Fast and the Furious sports car in your prime, shit can get hectic when you run like a Chevy Malibu as you age.

The thing is, a Chevy Malibu is a nice riding car, but it feels like garbage when you believe you were—and still should be—a Porsche 911. Speeding through this period of life like a Porsche Turbo S, and although at the moment it seemed like a blast, I clearly know now it took a toll on me mentally and emotionally.

By age 34, living a life that appeared on top of the world—with tons of women, money, cars, homes, and basically whatever I desired was attainable—but even with all of this, I felt empty and somewhat depressed. The momentary, instant gratification that came with a new material item or goal achieved was not improving my happiness.

And to make matters worse, every new woman I slept with made me feel worse and worse. Right after the enjoyable moment, I got emptier and emptier, to the point I knew I had to change. So in my mind, it was time to slow down and possibly settle down.

Easier said than done after a decade of entitlement and dysfunction. Trying to form a healthy relationship with a mindset of "my worth as a man is contingent on my finances and my dick." For many of us, that is the simple formula that validates you as a good man...simple as that.

The crazy part of it is, most men can feel validated by just one of the two. There are tons of men running around with complete acknowledgment they got wack dick, but because their finances and level of success are strong, they still feel like the man.

And on the flip side, some men are below-average earners, down to broke as a joke, but every time he slings some dick, he's got a three-orgasm minimum and you can't tell this brother shit. Now, in my case, I had both good dick and finances!

Now, what do both of these qualities get you? Entitlement like a motherfucker! Me, looking to settle down with a resume of good-looking, in shape, plenty of money, and good dick, was basically a blank check paid out to "have my cake and eat it, too."

In my mind, these two qualities were supposed to make any woman value me to the highest standard—and honestly, to most, it did. I was clearly considered a catch, and the women lined up. Fortunately, when you present your value to a woman as money and good dick, you get access to some of the most beautiful women available.

Unfortunately, the most beautiful women also have access to plenty of guys with money and good dick, too, so your sense of entitlement and validation is completely on thin ice. So my relationship at 32 was with a gorgeous girl who I had the emotion of love for, but when my shallow perspective of "I got money and good dick" wasn't enough to keep her away from other guys with money and good dick, I just fell deeper down the rabbit hole of disconnection.

She ended up leaving me for a basketball player on the New York Knicks, who clearly had way more money, and I guess I can safely assume…good dick. Not to mention, I'm a diehard Knicks fan with season tickets, so I ended up at games cheering for the guy my girl left me for. Can you say, "EMOTIONAL DAMAGE?"

Instead of being able to understand that it takes more than money and good dick to be truly a valuable man to a woman, I just chalked it up to "I must need MORE money and good dick" to validate myself as a man.

I was completely stuck in this formula that society sets as the precedent for a partner, and I was blind to any other way. The message is so strong that even women are being brainwashed into equating their value to this formula. It's all too common to hear single women reference their beauty and financial success as the deciding factor that determines if they are a good woman or not.

The relevance of this story is, although my example is on a higher level—maybe financially than the norm—men on every level equate a great portion of their value to money and good dick. It's the backbone of our validation system.

Society tells you that these two qualities are essential to finding and being successful with a mate. So it's no surprise that men who feel they are operating below standards as a provider are filled with tons of stress and feelings of inadequacy. But hopefully, you can fall back on your dick…

But God forbid the financial stress, or the decline in age and health, affects your sexual performance. Take that away too, and now you feel like nothing. Your value is gone in your eyes. Some guys get lucky and have a loving, supportive woman to build them back up. But chances are, if you operated like me from the shallow place of those two qualities are all that mattered, then your woman may not see you any differently than you see yourself. So as you feel you are failing in these areas, she can't even help remove this shallow stigma that is a confidence and erection killer—because you can't identify with any other value past having money and good dick. So, all hope is lost.

I didn't realize this shallow outlook that I once perceived as a great advantage—my so-called position of power—would be the straw that broke my back and completely crashed my mental health to a place where all my value was snatched from me.

CHAPTER ONE

My Story: From Celebrity Stripper to Totally Stripped of Confidence

By age 36 and after almost 15 years of believing I was the man, my world started to come crashing down. After my last breakup, where my lady left me for a guy with more money, I took the remedy of "getting more money" to the tenth power. The quick fix was going to come through real estate investing.

By this time, I had two brownstones in Harlem, a 9,000-square-foot mansion in Boca Raton, Florida, another 5,000-square-foot home in Fort Lauderdale, Florida, and another 20 rental properties in Ohio for cash flow. The value of these properties was about $10 million.

Now, here's the sweetest part: I bought all my properties at a steal, so based on appraisals, I had at least $3 million in equity combined. I was sitting pretty, just waiting for the right time to cash out.

Lo and behold, a little thing called the mortgage crisis showed up, and all my properties went belly-up. My $3 million in equity quickly became $2 million upside down.

Being an investor with the sole purpose of "getting more money so a dude won't take your girl," I recklessly overleveraged. I became minimally liquid, and by the time it was all said and done, I was broke and short-selling all my properties just to get in the clear.

Remember, I'm a guy who operates on the premise that my value as a man is having money and good dick—in that order—and now the money is gone, and as far as I was concerned, so was half my value. My mental state was starting to spiral.

Frantically, I tried to come up with a plan to pick up the pieces, but found no quick fix.

Then, out of nowhere, my phone rang. It was a casting director for a TV show called "Megan Wants a Millionaire" on VH1. I had auditioned for another show a few years prior that I didn't make, but the casting director remembered me and my prosperous financial situation and selected me as a fit for the show.

To be on the show, you needed a net worth of at least $1 million—and ironically, I was currently broke. Luckily, I still had enough material assets to create the illusion of success. I drove a Bentley, had an elaborate home (although pending foreclosure), Rolex watches, and so on. So, I was able to qualify for the show.

I came up with a plan that, from the free TV exposure, I was going to use it to catapult my male dancer business and a few other ventures, and not only be back on my feet but also have national celebrity status. I could see the light at the end of the tunnel, and my formula of money and good dick was going to be back in full swing.

Now, of course, if I was going on national TV, I wanted to look my best, so I hired a trainer to fast-track me into shape. Because of the short turnaround time, the only way to get in shape that fast was to do some anabolic steroids to accelerate the process.

It worked like a charm, and I was in the best shape of my life. I filmed the first show, and things went so well that I got invited to do a second show. Things could not have been going any better! As soon as these shows aired, my life would be the best it had ever been.

Or so I thought.

While my first show was airing in its early stages, one of my castmates committed a heinous crime and murdered his newly wedded wife. A massive manhunt ensued, which resulted in him hanging himself in a hotel room.

His terrible act caused VH1 to pull the show off-air, and the negative press led to the production company's entire line of shows getting scrapped, destroying my chance at salvaging my financial situation.

Now, to prepare for these shows, I had done a steroid cycle to get in shape. This wasn't my first steroid cycle, but I had done all the other ones in my early to mid-20s. Sadly, no one told me that a steroid cycle in your late 30s could crash your testosterone to the point of no return.

After using those steroids, getting my dick hard and maintaining an erection without the use of Viagra or Cialis was impossible.

So there I stood—no money, and now no good dick! In about 12 months, I was completely stripped of my perceived value as a man. My level of depression and feeling defeated was a place I never even knew existed.

I had hit rock bottom and just wanted to find any way to hold the pieces together to find my way back up.

The relevance of this story is that a lot of us, after hitting rock bottom—especially at a later age—never truly return to a place of prosperity. You can go from a place of trying to live to just trying to survive, and the survival standards most of the time are extremely low.

Being at rock bottom humbled me to just wanting to have a life where I could just get by day to day and maybe connect with a woman from time to time and hope that this new weak dick was enough to make her happy.

But this low-standard outlook on life is never gratifying. You never truly feel like a man again. So many men, both single and in relationships, are living with an inner feeling of their value stripped away—either their earning potential doesn't empower them, or their sexual function robs them of the confidence to feel valued that way.

It's a low, sad, and lonely place to be.

It pretty much feels like trading in your Porsche 911 Turbo S for a Chevy Malibu with the check engine light on. You are never going to be enthusiastic about driving that Chevy. That's how many of us are going through life right now.

If you hit rock bottom in life and it still has you down on the canvas, I can't help you get up from a financial standpoint, but I may be able to get your dick back on the road again.

You just have to want to. Keep reading and never give up on yourself.

I certainly did for many years, as I accepted this new diminished version of myself as acceptable. And over the next 10 years, the constant struggle it created—because of not truly doing all I could to address the issue.

It's better to try everything you can to fix it, as opposed to living with the problem. That thinking just makes you a dickhead—and in my case, it made me one literally.

I'll explain this more in the next chapter.

30

Don't Be a Dickhead!

As I shared in the previous chapter, I was now in my late 30s, early 40s, trying to recover from rock bottom. A formidable plan was in place to get my finances on track by rebuilding my stripper business as a company instead of being centered around me as an individual, and I must say that it was going well...

But I couldn't say the same for my non-cooperative penis.

The truth was, by this time, I was completely dependent on Cialis or Viagra, and even if I popped a pill, there was no guarantee of success. I had pretty much just adopted a formula of: I'll just pop a pill and hope for the best.

Whatever your own dicktale is—and there are a million of them—I'm coming at you with my own stories of erectile dysfunction—the dreaded dick droop syndrome. We're going to get into all the ways your dick can fail you and what to do about it in the chapters ahead, but first, I want you to know how high I was flying before I hit the ground.

As I'm sure you heard earlier, I was a pretty badass dude in the male stripping scene. I was known as THE PUNISHER, and that persona was an intimidating BDSM character who could never fail.

Women LOVED HIM! I had a lot of female fans, and you won't be shocked to hear that some of them wanted me to fuck them.

Did I want to give some of them what they wanted? HELL TO THE YES.

Now, this persona is fantastic for a 24 to 32-year-old in his sexual prime with enough dick energy to take down a volleyball team, but at 40 to 44, with an iffy erection—it was just a bunch of pressure I didn't want.

So every weekend, I was in the club, with an all-you-can-eat pussy buffet constantly available, and I was constantly saying, "No thank you, I'm watching my calories." Because of the onset of ED, I went from a ravaging sexual beast to practically scared of pussy.

With this onset of ED, I had to be very picky. My dick still worked if the chicks were fine as fuck, but the smallest detail could've deflated me instantly—and who wanted to deal with the embarrassment of that?

I met the Dominican girls you'll hear about in this chapter in my early 40s. Truth be told, I'd been experiencing creeping symptoms of ED since my early 30s, and that's not uncommon. But like most young men, I ignored it and blamed it on circumstances.

The first time I lost my erection, I was wearing a condom. So I blamed it on the condom, of course, because it couldn't be me.

Later, I blamed my worsening ED on how dark it was in the room—"Can't keep my dick hard if I can't see." So after that, I always adjusted the light.

Then it seemed like it was happening during certain positions, so no more cowgirl. It seemed to have something to do with what I was wearing, so I made sure to always remove everything, especially my socks (guys—always remove your socks before sex no matter what—those things will kill your erection).

The sound on the TV distracted me.

The temperature was too warm.

You name it; it was the problem. Anything but the obvious: I was developing ED.

Next, I needed formatted sexual experiences for success. I needed oral to achieve an erection before intercourse; then I could do penetration. No suck, no fuck. Should have had that on a T-shirt.

These quirks began to affect my relationships in a disastrous way.

This denial went on and on, but at this point, I knew it was not the condom, the lights, the position, or my socks being on... It was just me and my confidence.

With this new awareness, I found a little formula with myself: if I could get confirmation of the woman being sexually satisfied at any point early in the session, it would give me a confidence boost—and my dick would work fine.

For example, if I started sex by eating pussy and the girl orgasmed, I would get a confidence boost and could get an erection, as the pressure appeared to be less since she already climaxed.

At least that's the story I told myself—and it worked for my dick, so I was rolling with it.

Now, this formula was working until I got into a room with two of the sexiest girls you've ever seen—and I fucking blew it.

Before ED happened to me, I had literally no idea how common it was. Because it was still a shameful secret for me, I accepted this patched tire formula of success through Cialis and affirmations.

I was in UTTER DENIAL of it and just took this weak, diminished version of myself as all good.

33

It took years and some drastic circumstances to proactively try and truly fix it. And damn, man—because of that, I missed out on a hell of a lot of good times.

Meet the First-Ever Human Dickicorn

Lots of men fantasize about that dream scenario where multiple smoking-hot girls are lusting for us—all at once. You, my friend, are the power tool, and they both need drilling! The fantasy is as common as 10 fingers and 10 toes. If you're part of the select minority to have experienced this dream come true, I applaud you.

I was lucky enough to have my shot at stud immortality, only to finish my moment on the top of Mt. Everest in the worst outcome ever—a dickhead.

Here's the story...

My boy and I met these two smoking-hot Dominican girls. It was a classic two-man takedown as we went back to one of the girls' places. He had the cousin Ericka, and I had Gabriella. After some drinks, my boy went into the room with the cousin, and I was with Gabriella on the couch, and it was time for some action!

Now, I take pride in my sexual performance, so I had to put it down. These girls were hot, so I needed to make a good impression!

Like most men with onset ED (aka my dick works but not as well as it used to), we become expert pussy eaters! I mean triple black belt Bruce Lee level. Just call me Bruce Lick, because it's serious skill here.

Expert pussy eating is a way to compensate for what's missing in your penetration performance, so we take pride in it. Also, it's a confidence booster—making her cum usually mentally affirms we did a good job and decreases the anxiety you feel when your erection is iffy.

So I went nunchuck tongue on her pussy… Bruce Lick at his finest!

It was, of course, amazing—as I consider myself a grandmaster in tongue kung fu, so my record of success is impeccable. After the masterful pussy-eating performance, my confidence soared.

The confidence (plus a Cialis) allowed my erection to be good to go, and I gave her the intercourse version of a Rodney King beating. When it was all said and done, who's the man? Me! That's who!

In fact, my display of sexual skill was so spectacular that she told her cousin about my talents. Now, the woman I was with was beautiful, for sure—but her cousin was—oh my God!

So the very next weekend, Gabriella came out to the club with her cousin, Ericka. Both women wanted to hang out with me afterward. Their body language made it clear they weren't interested in walking around downtown Manhattan all night.

Of course, I was open to the idea of hanging out. After all, they were two beautiful women, and I consider myself an opportunist!

After the club closed, we went to Erika's place, and there were no formalities as they immediately invited me into the bedroom. The bedroom was set up like a sleep-in sex toy store. I couldn't believe all the sexual knick-knacks and novelties used as décor.

Dildos, vibrators, and every sex toy imaginable were all over the furniture, nightstands, and bed—it seemed. Even fucking handcuffs! Erika was a freak. I was like, *holy shit!* MY FANTASY IS COMING TRUE. I'M ABOUT TO REACH THE TOP OF STUD MT. EVEREST!

Because of my previous masterful sexual performance she was told about by Gabriella, Erika said in a deep sexy Latin accent, "Hey, I want to watch you fuck her now!"

Ericka then aggressively grabbed me and Gabriella, and we all climbed into bed. It was a queen-size mattress, so we were close. They were lying side by side, and I was on top of Gabriella, perched like an eagle ready to attack.

They both were naked, hot, and horny, and the pressure was on. Ericka was looking from the side, touching herself while reaching over to her nightstand, trying to pick a sex toy to play with. Gabriella was laying there, legs open and ready, quietly whispering, "Gimme, Papi... I want it, Papi."

And me... I was fucking terrified! I had the performance anxiety from hell. My dick was nonexistent. I was softer than whipped cream. This can't be happening.

I played it cool on the outside, but on the inside, I was screaming like the kid from the movie *Home Alone*. If the saying "pressure busts pipes" was a person—I'm him.

I was in full-fledged panic mode now as the girls were clearly ready and wanting action. There was only one solution—I went back to old reliable. Bruce Lick and the nunchuck tongue... and boy was I *Enter the Dragon*. I was eating Gabriella's pussy like I was plugged into a power outlet!

The licks were at the speed of light. If I had a switch, it was on high/level 10/DEFCON 1 — or whatever the highest level humanly possible. I'm pretty sure there was a buzzing sound similar to a vibrator radiating from my cheeks.

After about five mins, she let out a werewolf howl as she came, and I could hear harp music playing in the background, as in my mind I was being anointed the KING of pussy eating!

I popped my head up from between her legs to admire my work as she lay there in exhausted ecstasy. Her legs were apart and limp like a grenade exploded in her vagina!

I got a confidence jolt, and my erection shot up, ready to roll. I slipped on the condom super fast, as time is of the essence with ED. *Use it before you lose it* is serious, as the slightest distraction could deflate you instantly.

I penetrated Gabriella, and she was loving it. Her moans and breaths were a crystal-clear indication that my dick was feeling fantastic!

Ericka was so turned on watching, she reached over and started playing with her cousin's tits… now she was sucking them! I was like, OH MY FUCKING GOD—this is AMAZING!

She then started yelling out instructions for how I was to fuck her.

"Turn her this way."

"Put her leg up."

"Slow down."

"Kiss her."

Etc., etc.

Now, this may sound hot and sexy, but this was beginning to become a big problem. Like I mentioned earlier, erections with onset ED can be very tricky.

Playing her sexual Simon Says was starting to affect my erection. She was giving me way too much to think about, and my tire was going flat.

I was staying focused, and my thought process was: *As long as I'm in the pussy, creating stimulation… I should be alright!*

Then, out of nowhere, Ericka said, "I want it NOW, Papi! You come to me."

She aggressively pulled me right off and out of Gabriella and on top of her. I felt like a ragdoll the way she manhandled me. I was on top of her now, and she was telling me, "Change the condom, Papi, and give it to me… I want it so bad, Papi, please!"

I snatched off the condom as the clock was ticking. My erection outside of a vagina was like a vampire in sunlight… It was going to disintegrate.

I started frantically looking for the condoms—and these fuckers were nowhere to be found. They were mixed up in the bedding, and it was like a scavenger hunt to find them.

As I was looking, my anxiety was climbing, and my boner was dying. "NOOO, please, this can't be happening."

I finally found the condoms, which was about 30 to 45 seconds later, but in "*maintain your erection*" time, that is 1 hour and 24 mins. So my dick was as flat as a pita.

Fuck! I couldn't do anything and she was ready!

So, of course, what came to mind? Bruce Lick and my nunchuck tongue!

I dropped down between her fucking thighs and went to work, eating her out power-outlet style! Cheeks buzzing!

"No, Papi, I don't want that," she said. "I want you."

I was acting like I didn't hear her, still eating that pussy, arms locked around her thighs like a bungee cord harness.

"Come on, Papi. Come on, Papi. I want you now, Papi!"

Fuck that. I kept licking. I was determined to make her cum nunchuck tongue style—plus, my dick wasn't hard. I needed something to save me from failure.

While I wrestled with her thighs, trying to maintain my eating position, I felt a hard bop on the top of my head.

I thought she had hit me. *What the fuck happened? Did this girl just hit me?*

I popped my head up from between her thighs. "What the fuck was that?"

The minute they made eye contact with me, Erika and Gabriella let out hysterical laughter. I'd never heard anyone laugh this hard before. They were laughing so hard, they were gripping their stomachs, and tears were running down their flushed faces. Hugging each other, every time they looked at me, they laughed harder.

The top of my head ached. "What the fuck is so funny? What was that?"

They didn't answer. They just kept laughing, damn near rolling off the bed in hysterics.

I reached up and felt the top of my head. I felt the base of something. As I moved my hand up, it felt rubbery. It felt like a dick.

This woman had slammed a huge suction dildo to the top of my bald head. She grabbed it from the nightstand and suctioned it to the top of my fucking head.

"What in the fuck is this?" I asked them, but they were laughing so hard, they seemed in pain from laughing.

39

I got up and went to the mirror. A fucking big-ass, clear-colored, veiny dildo was stuck to my head! It was the type made to be mountable to the wall or any flat surface—and my bald head was prime for sticking.

To make matters worse, I couldn't get it off. It was stuck tight as hell. As I pulled, it felt like the skin was going to come off my head. I mean, Super Glue level.

How was I going to get this shit off my head?

Just snatching it off was not an option, so I changed the technique. I started pulling it lightly up and down, hoping to loosen it. Then I tugged with a little more tempo. I tried single-handed, then double-handed, just trying to find a way to get it off.

I noticed, as I was trying different techniques to get it off, the girls were laughing harder and harder, like they couldn't breathe. My different approaches to remove it looked like I was giving the dildo a fucking skilled hand job with a variety of hand strokes.

Like the dildo on my head was an overhead shake weight, and I was getting one hell of a workout.

They were near death from laughing… "This shit cannot be seriously happening."

That shit was so disrespectful. I just continued frantically pulling, trying to get that thing off my head. I was so pissed off. "How are you gonna do this to somebody?"

It didn't matter what I said; it fell on deaf ears as they were on the floor, crying with laughter.

In the midst of my anger and embarrassment, I stared at myself in the mirror. I took a long look at this huge dick dildo stuck to my head unicorn style and...

Eventually, I had to say to myself—*okay, this is some hilarious shit.*

It was hilarious. They won. I became the sexual version of a unicorn—the first-ever Dick-icorn.

Eventually, I got the dildo off my head, but there was no coming back from that.

So, I just left. Angry, embarrassed, and unfortunately a dickhead...literally.

So, the moral of this story is...don't be a dickhead. If I had addressed my onset ED issues instead of being in denial, I would have reached my Mt. Everest of sexual fantasy. So to all my brothers out there: you need to be proactive in fixing or preventing the ED problem. Learn from my pain or risk having an amazing sexual experience fall into your lap and miss out. Or worse, you could end up being a dick-icorn.

CHAPTER TWO

The Brain-Dick Pipeline: Fixing Your Mental Health Can Fix How You Feel About Your Cock

Why do so many of us men see our erections and sexuality deteriorate over time and do very little about it? Is there an unspoken understanding that, over time, our dicks are supposed to start acting up like a 10-year-old American car? "Goddammit, the check engine light is on again." If you have been one of these older car owners, like me, you know it's a love-hate relationship that is constantly hot and cold. One moment, you're praising the car for how good it's running, professing you are going to keep it forever. Then something goes wrong, and you're stuck on the side of the road, and you fly off the handle: "THIS PIECE OF SHIT CAR. THIS FUCKER'S GOT TO GO!"

Eventually, you get it to the shop and find out it's a $30 sensor and $150 to fix, and you think to yourself, "Well, that's not too bad." Now, your car is back on the road, and you're back to loving her and planning to keep her forever.

Then, at some point, breakdowns and car troubles become so frequent that you suddenly morph into a parking lot mechanic. Now you're pulling up to the repair shop, telling them, "You might want to check the throttle body or the MAF sensor; if neither one of those works, it could be the PCM." This up-and-down battle with keeping these old cars on the road is the same process we go through with our dicks when they start acting up.

We start out complaining and frustrated about the random breakdowns and run to our version of the local auto shop for a quick, inexpensive fix. When the problems continue, you jump online and read a few articles or forum threads to diagnose the issues. After you become savvy with that, you step it up and become your own dick's mechanic, changing oil, sensors, and brakes on your own after watching a few YouTube videos.

The truth is, you probably should see a high-level urologist or endocrinologist to give you an extensive workup to get to the root of the problem. But most of us see that as taking your 10-year-old car to the dealer for repairs. "Fuck that! The dealer is too fucking expensive!" So you go years and years doing what you can to keep your dick on the road. Sometimes it runs; others, not so much. But if the majority of the time she runs, you'll take it.

Shit, sometimes it's running great with the check engine light on, and you don't even take it to the shop, the light just goes off in a few days by itself. "Well, would you look at that?" At some point, we just accept our dick is a hooptie, and we are happy to just get from A to B.

I accepted my dick was a hooptie and knew exactly how to keep it running. I just had to warm it up for about 10 minutes, make sure the engine was nice and lubed, and keep the radio off because it drains the battery. Follow this formula, and my dick ran fine. But every now and again, out of the clear blue, my dick would run like a brand-new car fresh out of the showroom. "Where the fuck did that come from?" Let me tell you about the first time I experienced this and why I think it happens.

Freezer Meat in Paradise

When I was 38, I went to Turks and Caicos to visit a beautiful Albanian woman I'd met because I was dating her friend (yeah, yeah, I know, I ain't shit). We had been talking online for some time, and she finally invited me to visit. On the very first day on the island, she took me to this secluded private beach that was absolutely the most beautiful place I've ever been.

To this day, it's the closest I've been to paradise. Now, the coolest thing about this beach for me was that you could walk about a mile out into the water, and the current stayed as calm as a swimming pool, with the water never coming higher than your waist. I didn't even know something like this existed, and it was pivotal for me because I am the poster child for the stereotype, "Black people can't swim." Shit, I hold my nose in the shower... seriously.

So, we were about a quarter of a mile out, just in the water talking, laughing, and vibing, and I was totally immersed in this moment. Although this was our first moment together, it felt like we'd known each other forever. My mind was completely locked into the now and completely at ease. In a brief moment of tranquil silence, she turned toward me, hugged me, and straddled her legs around my waist. We immediately started to passionately kiss.

The moment was the equivalent of an award-winning romantic love scene from a movie. I mean, everything was storybook. This tall, handsome, muscular man embracing this gorgeous woman with hair flowing in the wind and water glistening all over her body—literally a scene you dream about that only happens in movies and romance novels.

It was clear the moment was right; the sexual tension was building, and she wanted me right then, right now! She reached down between her straddled legs and started to passionately undo the strings on my swim trunks. I immediately assisted by sliding my trunks down to mid-thigh, giving her unobstructed access.

She gazed straight into my eyes with an intense stare, took hold of my manhood, and let out a sigh of ecstasy before uttering the words that, to this day, made that moment the best sexual experience of my life. My fantasy, paradise moment culminated with, "Goddamn, this motherfucking dick feels as hard as freezer meat!" I instantly became overjoyed with emotion!

My exterior response was to stand there stoically, gazing off into the horizon like some sort of medieval world-conquering king before battle, who just flew in on a fire-breathing dragon with an army of 50,000 of the deadliest warriors behind him. Stud muffin on 10! But my inner response, on the other hand, was a flamboyantly gay hip-hop dancer doing the running man while uncontrollably giggling. I struggled to contain myself, as every part of me wanted to respond with, "Giggle, who? Me? Oh, stop it," as I blushed, "I bet you say that to all the guys." Giggle, giggle.

By this point in my life, I had been extremely successful and the top male stripper for about 15 years, so I had heard every form of compliment imaginable at least 20 times. I had reached a point where I was completely unfazed. "Yes, yes, I know I'm amazing... yes, thank you."

But calling my dick "freezer meat" while I was in the midst of struggling with ED was truly the most beautiful thing a woman had ever said to me. I tear up just thinking about it. Come on, bro! Do you know how fucking hard freezer meat is? We all know nothing hits harder (pun intended) than a dick compliment! This moment was the pinnacle of my erectile life. To recently be at rock bottom and bounce back with freezer meat is a hell of a comeback!

Like a lifelong politician starting as just the head of the neighborhood watch and getting elected president of the United States, it was completely unexpected, as my confidence in my erection had been fleeting for some time. Her resounding compliment about my dick being that hard took me by complete surprise. There was no way in my wildest dreams I expected that!

The only other time in my life I was that surprised was in 2016 as a Black man in New York City hearing the announcement that Donald Trump had won the election: "WAIT!"—clueless face—"That motherfucker WON?!"

At this time in my life, my erection had already been like a box of chocolates—"You never know what you're gonna get," (Forrest Gump voice)—and honestly speaking, the last thing I expected was freezer meat.

I rode that momentum, and for the rest of the trip, my erection was freezer meat all day, every day. We had effortless, amazing sex every day, and I was completely confused because my dick hadn't worked this well in years. Talk about my 10-year-old hooptie running like a brand -new car. Truly baffled by the resurgence of my erection to its highest level, I eventually chalked it up to the Caribbean, telling all my friends, "Yeah, bro, that salt water and the extra vitamin D from the sun are like a battery boost for your dick."

This is why old dudes move to Florida — to get more dick sun! I was convinced that was the secret.

Now, there are some scientific benefits to climate-boosting libido, but to go from a gummy worm to freezer meat fresh off the plane is a stretch. I understand now that my erection resurgence was mental. Being completely present in that moment in paradise allowed me not to worry about the stress of my normal life.

More importantly, I had absolutely no expectations that we would have sex that afternoon in the middle of the water. It was truly the furthest thing from my mind, which was extremely helpful because my norm prior to sex would be to overthink, worry about my erection, performance, etc. The anxiety would hamper my ability to perform. This spontaneity and unexpectedness prevented me from getting in my head, which was essentially my own enemy.

The bottom line was that if I removed the stress and anxiety of the moment, my dick was fine. But instead of focusing on these mental aspects, I kept popping pill after pill, trying to fix a mental problem with a physical remedy. So if your 10-year-old hooptie of a dick, every now and then, runs like a brand-new car, the issue may not be the car, but actually the driver—aka YOU!

As for me, I didn't have a book to buy that pointed this out, so I just kept chasing the freezer meat high like a drug addict, going from dealer to dealer, hoping to replicate that wonderful day in the sun when my dick was at its greatest!

In the years that followed, whenever I felt stressed, anxious, or depressed about my flagging erection, I'd remember that once, back in the day, my dick was as hard as freezer meat. It was like a standard was set; it was the pinnacle I was always trying to get back to.

I've often joked, "It was all downhill from there!" as I could never quite make it back to freezer meat status. But why was it so important to me? At the time, I was having good sex; the hooptie (my dick) was riding nice with minimal problems as long as I did the 10-minute warm-up, etc.

But I just couldn't shake the obsession with the need for freezer meat. I mean, years and years of chasing this result ultimately ended in me getting an implant. Why was I so obsessed with this goal? Because that moment, when I received that glorious praise about my amazing dick, was much more than the highlight of my sexual life—it was a reconnection to my masculinity. That was the high I was actually chasing.

As we know, masculinity is a lot of things, but you must admit that one of the ways our society measures masculinity is by a dick that's as hard as freezer meat!

So when I had that idyllic moment in the Caribbean, my mind, body, and soul understood it as the most affirming moment for my masculinity ever. Not because it actually was, but because nothing feels more emasculating than prolonged suffering with ED.

That moment reconnected me with feeling like the man I was, like the man I wanted to be. No matter how I excelled in other aspects of life, I just couldn't truly feel good about myself with a dick that had the check engine light on.

Is that the main component of my masculinity? Probably not. But that didn't stop me from thinking about it relentlessly.

My thoughts on *What's wrong with my dick?* began casually and then became a fixation over years. I only realized how much I'd been obsessively thinking about my boner (aka, my missing boner) after I got my implant, and it was no longer on my mind all the time. I was like, holy shit, imagine everything I could've accomplished if I hadn't spent the last decade obsessively worrying about my dick.

It took way too long to get to where I am now—a life-changing implant—which is a great place to be, to be honest. It didn't have to take so long for me, and it doesn't need to take that long for you, either.

Looking back, it is clear to me that my dick became an influence on every part of my life. Every action I made seemed to have a direct correlation to my dick. Slowly but surely, if I worked out, it wasn't to look good anymore; it was "got to raise my testosterone for my dick."

The foods I was eating were "got to eat these foods for my dick." Every vitamin or supplement became "I need these for my dick."

If I was out and about and being flirted with by a nice girl, I'd think, *Can't talk to her. My dick might not like her.* I became a complete mental case trying to deal with this dick obsession. It was on my mind all the time and had crept into every aspect of my life.

Take a minute to ponder it: how many times a day do you think about your dick? Be honest with yourself. And not in the stereotypical way that people say, "Men think with their dicks." I'm not talking about being horny or thinking about sex. I'm talking about worrying about your dick.

Whether you're thinking about its size, how hard you got the last time you were in a sexual situation, how long or short it takes you to cum, or whether your partner likes it or not—

you're probably thinking about your cock's functioning a bit too much.

Just sit here for a minute and estimate how much time per day you're thinking about your dick. Ten minutes? Thirty minutes? An hour? All fucking day long?

This constant concern is when the anxiety starts to grow, which eventually becomes an absolute erection killer. But the deeper truth is that it's not really about your erection. We've all had plenty of sex, and half of you reading this are probably at home right now with an accessible vagina in the form of a wife or girlfriend that you barely want to touch.

This is not about sex; it's about the masculine identity that often feels incomplete for many of us without a dick we can feel proud of.

The Hardest Question: What in the Actual Fuck is Masculinity?

But seriously, what is masculinity, for real? Men are so fucked up about this idea that they start wars (see Napoleon), and women are so confused about this idea that they don't understand men and what we need, putting a lot of pressure on us to live up to societal standards (see every relationship you've probably ever been in and several chapters that follow this one).

When I tell you that mental health is the bridge to curing erectile dysfunction, what I'm really talking about is our relationship to the concept of masculinity.

I'm what you may consider in this day and age 'old school' when it comes to masculinity. For me, masculinity can mean lots of things, but these are my top eleven:

1. Confidence
2. Independence
3. Responsibility
4. Honesty
5. Purposefulness
6. Leadership
7. Integrity
8. Assertiveness
9. Logic
10. Emotional intelligence
11. Strength (physical capability)

Notice that I didn't include any dick-specific qualities on this list. That's because masculinity goes way beyond your dick. But even with that understanding and my own list of masculine qualities not including dick qualities, absolutely nothing affected my masculinity like onset ED.

It made me fragile. I may have appeared tall and strong on the outside, but inside, I felt weak. More so in the moments of failure, when my erection let me down, I felt completely emasculated.

I would hide behind lies most of the time, such as, "I'm just really stressed over work" or my go-to, "I did legs at the gym, and the pain in my legs is just too unbearable." If you can relate to this, you have to really ask yourself: are you chasing just the ability to have sex? Because that's an easy fix. But if you're chasing the salvation of your masculinity, this problem may not be solved with just a boner.

Andrew Tate and the "Masculinity Movement"

We live in a time where, out there on social media, there's a divide between misogynists and feminists. The voice of "the men" has become represented by guys like Andrew Tate and Kevin Samuels, along with the whole "red pill awareness." There's this message that men should be masculine and return to our power and strength by being leaders and providers and putting our foot down with our women partners.

It's a very controversial message, and many feminists—perhaps even your own wife or girlfriend—believe guys like Andrew Tate and these other characters are total shitbags and they hate their guts. Yet thousands and thousands of men idolize this message, not just because they agree with it, but because they need something like this. They're lost, trying to figure out how to create value for themselves and function in this world.

You know what? There's a place and time where a lot of that applies. I don't agree with one side or the other—each to their own—but what I will say is that one conversation that's not happening in this whole "masculinity movement" is addressing erectile dysfunction and the huge part it plays in this message.

The men in their sexual prime and capable lovers obviously don't need this discussion, but I know a lot of men who are quietly struggling with their sexual abilities while overlooking the fact and latching on to the message from guys like Tate, which essentially says that money, status, and power are the keys to women and masculinity. Yet, all around us, we see some of the richest, most powerful men consistently failing at relationships. According to the standards of these men, they are the epitome of masculine/high-value men.

There has to be something missing in this message.

Now, I could delve into a host of reasons why this may be happening, but this is a book about dicks, so I'll stick to the point.

When a man doesn't feel like a man, it has nothing to do with money, status, career, or "putting your foot down." It's often about your inability to perform. I'll prove it to you. If you had a choice between money, status, career, and "putting your foot down," but your dick didn't work at all, would you take that deal? Or, on the flip side, how about living a below-average, humble life regarding status, money, and career but having everyone you have sex with get the best experience of their lives, and you would go down as their greatest lover until the end of time?

Now, how about that deal? I don't know about you, but I'm going with Option B. Yeah, I know those two hypotheticals are extreme, but it's to make an extreme point. There's only so far you can get in the masculinity conversation if you are limited in your sexual function.

A lack of intimacy caused by an inability to perform can plague our sense of self. The fear of not being sexually potent creates a dark cloud and a state of depression, triggering all sorts of anxiety. This is what makes many men feel devalued and full of shame.

That, to me, is the backdrop of a lot of the issues men are turning to Tate's message to cure. Because no one wants to talk about it—about their struggles with intimacy and performance issues—and they try to remedy it with the band-aid of money, status, and influence.

And when that doesn't work, or if his earning potential doesn't allow him to, he'd rather just blame society or women for his problems. "These bitches ain't shit!" This is a silent cry in the dark that is playing out in society, especially in my age group (over 40) and among the majority of my peers.

Now, don't get me wrong. I'm not saying everyone my age is running around with dick problems. I'm just reverting to the concept I spoke about earlier, where my value as a man was purely contingent on money and the benefits that came with it, along with having good dick. Today's message about masculinity is completely centered around the money/ power aspect and does not address the elephant in the room for men who are struggling sexually.

So even if a guy wanted to listen to Andrew Tate, proclaiming, "I'm gonna be the man and make all the money, make decisions, and lead my woman on the highest level," based on this guidance, how do you achieve that full level of masculinity when you can't even get your dick hard?

Can you truly feel masculine or apply any of those teachings? Can you really engage with any of the messages in society today if you are operating from a place where you can't perform sexually for your woman?

A lot of times, our ladies are actually fine with what they get sexually, but if you are not confident, how can you truly feel a part of the masculinity movement? The standard societal expectations are so high that very few can live up to them, yet the message targets the majority.

To put it in context, Tate's red pill message is equivalent to the NBA. Their playbook will definitely help you win the game of masculinity if you are an NBA player in life. The problem is, there are only 450 players in the NBA, but millions of guys playing basketball. So, no matter how good Tate's coaching is, if your life doesn't translate to being 6 feet 8 inches and 250 pounds like LeBron James, you can't apply the coaching Tate gives.

Every other day, I'm on the phone with one of my broke 40+ friends, dependent on Viagra, talking about, "I'm going to use this turnaround fadeaway jump shot I learned from Tate on these hoes…"

And I'm thinking to myself, *Dude, in life, you're not an NBA player. You're playing high school JV, and you're 5 feet 6 six and 145 pounds. Those moves aren't working for you!*

So when his shot gets punched into the stands because a fadeaway doesn't really help a 5-foot-6 guy, he blames it on women. This could possibly be the "toxic masculinity" that women are complaining about—where you're expressing your frustrations and fears and projecting your own lack of ability onto women. This is a very dysfunctional way to hide from your personal issues.

You can embrace the concept and practice of masculinity if you're operating from a place of confidence with mental and physical wellness—where all of your boxes are checked.

I personally struggled with my masculinity over a long period because of my inability to perform sexually and maintain an erection, even though I had money, career, and status. None of that matters if you are dealing with a lack of confidence.

So a natural reaction would be to make up for your financial or sexual issues in other ways, right? But unfortunately, you have guys like Tate and the red pill community ridiculing men for trying to compensate for their lack of confidence, calling them "simps." The level of irresponsibility to tell men who are trying to overcompensate for their shortcomings through pedestaled treatment of women is a terrible message to broadcast to the masses.

I do agree that there is a percentage of women who find it hard to respect men who fit any kind of "simp" definition and will never reciprocate the same interest or feelings. The message of simping is becoming twisted among the masses; the pedestaled treatment of any woman, whether she is mutually interested or not, is a no-go.

I believe the majority of women appreciate what's deemed "simping," as it can be a benefit for most guys.

More importantly, for a lot of guys, it's just not possible to operate from a strong position of power that Tate promotes because, as I mentioned earlier, they are simply not NBA players in life—no matter how much they try to be.

So simping, as it's defined, is all they have. To me, it's only an issue if your simping emasculates you or damages your confidence more—which happened to me (I will touch on this in "My Shitty Story").

To be clear, it's easy to follow society's protocol for masculinity if you are strong in both financial and sexual positions. But what do you do if you're not? That certainly puts you in a pickle! Instead of accepting this fate, why don't you do all you can to fix your pickle? At least half of the problem will be solved; I'm just saying.

Now, I operate from a place of confidence in my sexuality—and I've never felt more like a man.

You can feel completely whole again as a man and truly embody masculinity without following Andrew Tate's YouTube channel. Let's get real about this: blaming your masculinity issues on women is bullshit. I did this—I blamed my issues on the women in my life. But it was me all along.

So even though it's not ideal that society forces us into the uncomfortable position of needing to be masculine to feel good about ourselves, it is what it is. It's the hand we've been dealt as men, and maybe down the line, things will be different for your grandkids, but as of now... it's your money or your dick, and without one or the other, you ain't shit.

Erectile Dysfunction is Crippling Dudes Everywhere
I want to dive into the many ways we are affected beyond just having an erection for sex and the loss of confidence. Things start off small but can easily fester into much bigger issues mentally and create a cycle that is hard to get out of. Erectile dysfunction is a mental health problem that is crippling men everywhere, and in many ways, it's because we've lost sight of all the ways we can (and must) reconnect to our masculinity.

ED creates all kinds of severe mental and emotional issues for men, not just physical ones. Complicating matters, some mental health issues cause ED.

Depression
Many studies show that there is a clear link between ED and depression. In some cases, depression can cause ED. In other cases, ED can cause depression. But they are definitely entangled, and if you suffer from either, you should explore

the links and address them. Letting either ED or depression fester, even separately, can lead to a much bigger problem. Yes, there are a lot of drugs for depression, sometimes called SSRIs, but they can cause ED. So if your doctor prescribes them to cure your depression that you originally developed because of ED, you should have a long talk about avoiding options that cause or exacerbate performance issues.

Anxiety

Anxiety and depression are often two sides of the same coin. If you're feeling depressed some or all of the time, you probably also experience anxiety. Where depression can make us want to hide out in bed and do nothing, anxiety hypes up our nervous system and makes us hypervigilant. Sometimes, you can have anxiety without accompanying depression. The good news is that when anxiety is the main cause of your erectile dysfunction, there is a lot you can do to fix that shit. From cognitive behavioral therapy (CBT) to breathing exercises, meditation, and other techniques that don't require medication, it's one of the most "curable" forms of mental health issues.

Sexual performance anxiety is a subset of other kinds of anxiety, and it can get so intense that it may seep into other areas of your life, causing you stress. Needless to say, this SUCKS and nipping it in the bud early is your best bet.

Stress

This is just regular life shit—money problems, relationship issues, parenting problems, divorced parenting problems, dealing with aging parents' issues, work problems—the list goes on. If something is bothering you in your life at large, that issue can creep into your bedroom and kill your erection.

Relationship Stress

This is a very specific kind of boner-killing stress that's a subset of regular stress. If your relationship is on the rocks, it can affect your dick. Even if you're in a new relationship and you're super horny for each other, the stress of caring so much about a new partner and wanting to impress her can still affect your dick. If you're being nagged, that can affect your dick. If you think your partner is cheating, it can affect your dick—the list is endless.

This is why it's ALWAYS NECESSARY to start communicating clearly and honestly with your lover, no matter what stage your relationship is at. Your best bet? Start this shit at the BEGINNING. Chapter Eight is all about how to do this.

Sometimes, you can have a temporary physical impairment, something as simple as not getting enough sleep the night before, having COVID (which causes ED, dudes—avoid this illness at all costs), or some other minor problem that causes your erection to falter once or twice. But because we're so much more sensitive than we'll ever admit, guys will take this small, temporary incident and blow it up in their minds, causing a spiral of actual, ongoing erectile dysfunction.

There are more serious physical issues that can cause ED—issues that you definitely need to discuss with your doctor.

• High blood pressure

- Heart disease
- Obesity
- High cholesterol
- Sleep disorders
- Parkinson's disease
- Alcoholism
- Low testosterone (more on this in a later chapter)

I dealt with ED for years, and every time I went to the doctor, I got a completely clean bill of health. This is very common, because, as I said, most dick problems are in your head. That's good news, fellas, because we can fix what's in our heads by making a few tweaks. Relationships are a great place to start tweaking. But you have to be proactive and motivated to make changes.

Many of us are sitting with these issues plaguing our relationships and doing nothing about it—or, even worse, doing things that just make the situation worse.

CHAPTER THREE

Unshaming Your Shaft: Making Space For Vulnerability With Erectile Dysfunction

When Everything Fell Apart... My Shitty Story

As I touch on throughout the book, psychogenic ED is something that grows in your mind over time. For me, the seeds were planted in my teens, and life circumstances watered them to a point where they were ready to bloom like gardens in the spring. Up to this point, I had been holding on to some great sexual function and a decent degree of confidence until I got involved with the relationship that would be the nail in my coffin.

Some years ago, before I got my implant, I ended up in a long-term relationship with a married woman who was in a sexless marriage. She had been married for seven years, had four children, and at some point, she and her husband had a complete disconnect sexually.

That disconnect happened ironically because her husband couldn't perform. He developed Peyronie's disease (also called penile fibrosis), which is the curvature of the penis that can create erection issues. Having sexual issues (which he never communicated directly about because we're all told not to be vulnerable) made him turn a blind eye to his woman sleeping with other men, seeking her satisfaction elsewhere. For a lot more men than you think, it's easier to let your girl fuck other guys than to talk about your dick problems.

While he acted not exactly as if nothing was wrong, he molded their marriage into more of a roommate-friendship scenario. This caused a lot of tension, friction, and negativity—and they barely spoke. However, he had written up an agreement he emailed to her, which she showed me, allowing her to seek other relationships. He, too, could do the same as long as they respected the boundaries of their relationship, their neighborhood, and that they upheld the appearance of their marriage. When she showed me this email, it was the green light for me to get involved in this situation.

In the beginning, I was only in it for a good time, no ties. Since she was married and occupied, my involvement was straight about sex—nothing more, nothing less. Get a hotel room once a week, meet her there, put in my Bruce lick, have a little batting practice, and walk out of there feeling like "the man." This went on for some time.

At the onset of my ED, it was very important for me to get sexual validation because I was very insecure about my masculinity. So, I went into every sexual situation trying to be the best lover possible. It was important to me to be affirmed and acknowledged this way because, deep down inside, although I was in denial, I knew I wasn't at my best. But hey, what I put out could have still been all good to somebody, and that's what I needed to hear and feel when dealing with my sexual partners.

So, I showed up every week and put in the work. This married woman let me know she had been aware of me for years. I told you that I was a very popular male stripper in New York City —and well, she was a fan who traveled from

62

show to show to see me. Somehow, I'd never met her even though she was always there in the crowd. She had a huge infatuation with me—I was like her dream guy, and this was extremely flattering.

In my mind, this woman had been scouring the Earth to get my dick. It was amazing! Talk about an ego boost! So, I took part in her fantasy and became her "dream come true," according to her. This woman was extremely affirming because everything about our sex was amazing to her—she reacted like it was the greatest experience ever.

Now, this response and expression from her was detrimental. As a man with diminishing sexual ability, I lived with a sense of intense insecurity. The emphatic expression of her satisfaction was so profound and positively impactful on my self-confidence that I was on a high I hadn't felt in years. It was everything my ego needed as a man in terms of the way she treated me and the way she responded sexually—everything was at its peak.

It wasn't quite a "freezer meat" moment, but it was close.

So, this affair went on for several years, and for what it was worth, I found myself in a full-fledged relationship with this woman, with feelings, attachments, and everything you would expect, but it was a one-sided scenario. She was married; I was single, and there wasn't much that she could offer me in this part-time scenario. Honestly, though, it didn't matter.

Coming into this situation, I was a broken man. Between the unhealed trauma of a previous heartbreak, stress about the uncertainty of my future goals, and the onset of my sexual decline, I was full of fear and insecurities that had me avoiding close relationships for the previous twelve years.

My heart was a vault, and no one was getting in. I would come into situations with the lowest expectations and standards. It was a foregone conclusion that everyone was going to cheat, lie, deceive, and hurt me.

I just accepted that it was going to happen and became mentally and emotionally prepared for more damage. I was so hurt that I was essentially starting relationships with that "turning a blind eye" theory. Loyalty was not an expectation at all, and the best I could hope for was honesty.

To get the honesty, I would paint myself as extremely understanding so my partner could come to me and tell me anything. As long as it came from her, it would be fine.

Mentally, this was a way to avoid being blindsided by hurtful information, which fueled my relationship trauma. It was a terrible way to look at relationships, but it felt one hundred times safer than being vulnerable.

I was very transparent with this married woman about my outlook. She was a therapist by trade, so she completely understood and shared that she, too, had been hurt in similar ways. She was adamant in affirming I could trust her, she was different, and she wanted no one else. We then put agreements in place that we would be honest with each other.

We agreed the thing that hurt the most was being blindsided. We said everything would always be on the table. We would be the different person in each other's history. We would heal each other. I bought completely in. It was everything I wanted to hear. I needed that. I needed her.

So, the fact that she was married and had no intentions of leaving didn't matter. I was willing to settle for what she provided on a part-time basis. I only had one stipulation.

Because she had no intention of leaving her marriage, it was only fair that I had a window of opportunity. Meaning, if I met someone with whom I could build a family and future, I could kick the tires on its potential.

She said, "It would hurt to lose you, but I believe you deserve a wife and family of your own." She just wanted me to be upfront and honest with her so she wouldn't be blindsided. Which, of course, I wouldn't have had it any other way.

I appreciated her consideration of my need for flexibility, and I put my "turn a blind eye" offer on the table to give her the option to do what she wanted outside of us. I proposed I would only focus on our time together, and what she did outside of us was her business. That suggestion received a resounding, "Absolutely not!"

She emphatically explained, "I am a one-man woman. I am completely committed to you and only you!"

She even said she would not deal with anyone and did not want nor need consent. I even pushed for her to agree, as this was also for my own personal safety.

I had put these dysfunctional terms on the table to keep my walls up and expectations low. However, she would have none of it. She only had eyes for me.

"So, let me get this straight. You're giving me a free pass to find my possible wife and you're still going to be completely devoted to me?" At that moment, my free pass was moot. Where was I going to find another amazing woman like this?

Let me tell you. Being in an insecure, doubtful place as a man, to have had a woman come along and affirm me like that, it was life-changing. She pulled me right out of the gutter, so to speak, and placed me on a throne. Married or not, I was not letting her go.

After four years, she started pursuing a divorce to open the door for us to have a more significant relationship other than my just being a glorified side guy. For a long time, she had desired for us to have a closer, loving relationship, but her marriage always was a sticking point that limited our growth. There was only so much, with my traumatic history, she could have gotten from me as a side guy.

I wouldn't have been able to fully invest until she was free, and now she was willing to make it happen.

This was a great thing for me because I completely trusted her, which was unheard of for me. She had built up my self-esteem so that I was in the best place I could be. Finally, I felt valued again—something I had given up on years ago. A feeling I desperately needed, and for this, she was truly everything to me.

Now, during this time, things weren't perfect. We had a mishap where she went to a "so-called" training event for one of her sex therapy courses. One thing led to another, and she ended up cheating on me. I found out by asking her an honest question, to which she admitted.

As I said, I make safe places for partners to come clean. I was extremely hurt, and we had broken up, but eventually, my turn-a-blind-eye ways crept in, and I forgave her. I sold myself on self-blame, and to be honest, she had contributed so much to building my confidence, I didn't want to let her go.

She adamantly apologized, blaming the terrible decision on doubts about how I felt about her, which I understood because I'm not the most verbally expressive. She assured me nothing like that would ever happen again.

After patching it up, and a year later, I started to question if she was truly the loyal, devoted woman she claimed to be.

As a male stripper, there are inherent complications because of my workplace circumstances. When you're in an environment where bachelorettes and married women in the club are going crazy, and interacting inappropriately with you and your coworkers, it messes up your trust and belief in that system.

The woman I was dealing with had a highly sexualized nature, plus she had already admitted to cheating on me. I began questioning some things throughout our relationship, even though I had full trust in her. So, I hit her with something a lot of couples do.

"Hey, look, if we're gonna take the next step, let's not have any secrets, any baggage, anything in the closet that we didn't reveal to each other."

We had a heart-to-heart, open conversation about whether she was being completely honest and if I had been as well. We were going to put it all out on the table.

So, for three weeks, we had conversations, and I disclosed whatever went on while we were together, and she gave me about seven different scenarios with different men. "Oh, I went on a date with this guy," "I hung out with this guy," and "I gave this guy my number," but with all these situations, none of them ended up with her having sex with anybody or anything significant happening, so she said.

Since I've been around the block and realized that when people tell lies, they give you 90% of the truth, and they just leave out the 10% they know that's going to piss you off, all the information is pretty accurate, but they know what not to say.

I questioned her for three weeks and got all the information I wanted—or so I thought. Her story was changing every other day. She was clearly making stuff up. So we finally got to where she said, "And now you know everything."

These days, we should ideally be able to back up our stories with text messages, phone records, photos, and some sort of correspondence to match up with the interactions and the information. Ironically, everything that happened in these situations, she just happened to have deleted from her phone. How convenient.

"Oh, I don't like stuff on my phone. I need to keep my storage," she said, along with the bullshit reasoning of why there was no information available on the phone.

So, no problem. I just pulled one of my Jedi mind tricks. I said, "Listen, on the dark web, there are these programs that you can get. They're usually used by law enforcement because criminals keep evidence on their phones, and then they try to delete it when they get caught.

"So the police and the FBI can put these special programs on your phone to retrieve all your messages, photos, and emails. You know, AT&T, T-Mobile, Verizon, and all the carriers are aware of this. This is something they installed, so it's all still on your phone in a folder that you can only access with this program.

"I'm going to buy this program on the dark web, and we're gonna put it on your phone, so we can pull up all those messages because I believe you, but I just want to be sure."

I told this multi-degreed, therapist by trade Ph.D. professional, forty-something-year-old woman that I was going to do this, and she immediately spilled her guts.

"Okay. Okay. Okay. Okay. I fucked this one, I fucked that one," and the truth came out.

I will not make light of the story because it devastated the hell out of me. This was a woman I loved, a woman I fully trusted, and it was really hard to get to that point when I came into the situation already jaded with an extremely untrusting nature.

I was very transparent with her about my insecurities and the betrayals I'd experienced. She knew I didn't want to go through that again. As a therapist, she understood me from a clinical perspective and could break down my issues, my PTSD, my anxious-avoidant attachment style, and a bunch of other lingering traumas.

She assured me she was different, that I could trust her, that I had nothing to worry about, and that everything was going to be fine. She was the woman I needed; she was different, and I didn't have to worry about her, and it was all bullshit. I got the timeline.

I offered her consent to do whatever she wanted; she declined and insisted on being loyal to me. Affirmed to me practically daily on her being the woman I could trust to the point where a man that swore to never trust a woman again bought in completely... all the while she was fucking and sucking the whole time and in the most frivolous way.

Random guys that she would aggressively initiate, pay for the hotel room, and just do her. Don't get me wrong, I'm not trying to shame her for being an empowered woman and living her sexual life how she chose. My issue was this: why was it necessary to create and repeatedly affirm her loyalty when it was abundantly clear it was never her intention?

Especially knowing, on a clinical level, that she was dealing with a man who was doing everything in his power to avoid being betrayed again?

I already told you that my stage name is "The Punisher." I would come out on stage with the leather, the whips, the chains, exhibiting a whole BDSM vibe (erotic practices or roleplaying involving bondage, discipline, dominance, submission, and sadomasochism). This woman told me her interest in me was always about her fantasy and her curiosity about BDSM. She had hoped that when she met me, The Punisher was a true part of my sex life and that we would embark on a BDSM sexual relationship.

Now, I'm cool with BDSM, but it's not necessarily my sexual preference. It requires clear communication and boundaries—couples need to discuss it upfront. She had a great interest in this, but she never mentioned it to me.

She then told me that since I didn't initiate BDSM, and it was something she wanted to try, she needed to seek it behind my back! Basically, it was my fault, and that was bullshit. I think she just had some narcissistic tendencies, did her thing, and there was no accountability to be taken. So she cheated, and I was to blame.

She cheated on me with a BDSM porn star. Now, this guy was all over social media, all over the Internet, all over anywhere to be found. He had a gigantic fucking horse dick and she hired him. Now, while I was her man, giving her the best dick I had to offer, she was going out and buying a bigger dick on my watch.

Fellas, not only was she pursuing this bigger dick that she felt she needed to pay for, she was doing it in the BDSM mindset. So this guy had her on her knees, calling him her king, her master, spanking her, fucking her in the face, got a dog chain around her neck, barking orders at her she was obeying like a well-trained puppy, and proud of it.

So proud that she shared her infatuation with him with all her girlfriends and would pull up his videos on the regular at the bar and get-togethers to show him off to her crew.

All her close friends knew, and I was the idiot, thinking I was special. Mind you, this guy was married with a child and couldn't offer her anything other than a sexual moment she had to pay for, but it was clear he was the object of her desire.

My time as the love object was over. She inquired how she could create a long-term, paid situation with him. She asked to be his first call when he came to town to ensure she was the first to get the dick before it got dirty from other local customers. Basically, she needed a side guy for her side guy. Just for sex, I guess?

Well, my self-esteem was in the toilet. She was open with telling me he was a better lover than me because of his BDSM and said it was the biggest dick she had ever had, while letting me know my sex had become "too routine," was only good "every other time," and "your dick doesn't get as hard as it used to," were just a few of the inadequacies that she claimed led her astray.

Ironically, amid this admittance, he texted her to let her know he and his dick were coming to her area. She shared this with me, and I asked her to cut it cold.

71

I told her specifically, "Text him back and tell him I will no longer be in need of your service. Please don't text me anymore." I thought this was a more than reasonable request.

However, she refused, saying, "I don't want to rudely cut him off like that. I'm grateful for the time with him, so I'm not going to be rude."

Grateful? My woman was grateful for some guy letting her buy his dick in a hotel room she paid for and fucking her like a stray dog? Could it have gotten any worse? Actually, yes!

A few weeks prior to her first time seeing him was my girl's birthday. From the time I met her, she spoke of this Chanel dress she just loved. The dress was discontinued and not available anywhere. I scoured the Earth, and I found it at a Kim K celebrity auction. I outbid everyone and got it for her for $5,000.

She was so happy, which made me happy. I was so proud to have gotten that for her. She made it clear she cherished the dress and couldn't wait to wear it. So when was the first time she wore it? To go see the guy she was paying to fuck her! She wore my gift to look good for him. Even sent me selfies on her way to meet him. Like a true dumbass, I complimented how amazing she looked in it!

This was emotional damage on a catastrophic scale for a man who, at some point, felt that he was his woman's Mount Everest of sex.

Her affirming all of this to me, only to find out that she was buying dick and submitting herself to another man on this type of level, and to blame my inadequacy as her motivation, was a dick killer. After all the years of decline, the end of this relationship just amputated it.

I was done. This shattered my ego, shattered my confidence, shattered everything that I still held about maintaining myself as a lover. Finding out about this situation and the details she vividly shared with me when she thought I was going to look at her phone… it was too much.

That was it for me. I went from somebody with an early onset ED, still functioning pretty well and feeling confident, to not being able to achieve an erection at all for months. It was just devastating.

It was all I could think about. It was a ruminating thought, a constant issue for me, mentally and emotionally. I was experiencing a deep form of betrayal trauma. I had PTSD from that situation. Everything reminded me of her with him. It fucking consumed me to no end.

I even started watching his porn videos constantly as some form of exposure therapy. I bought books on BDSM, whips, floggers, and a host of other kinky shit. In my mind, and based on what she had told me, I needed to be a better lover. I listened to her, and I blamed myself and my inadequacies. I went on a quest to correct myself by any means necessary.

I visited countless doctors to consult about procedures to improve my erection, make my dick bigger. Hell, I tried every ED drug/supplement I could find. My level of desperation was clear mental illness.

During this time, she was supportive as she could be, and I wanted to believe she was remorseful. I tried to create sexual BDSM experiences for her, as this was the sex life she wanted, and the whole time I was tormented.

I could no longer be present with my own sexual enjoyment, as the pressure and anxiety to do a good job was all I cared about. At that moment, I would envision her with him, and it was a constant comparison in my mind.

I studied BDSM like a law student preparing for the bar exam, and I can honestly say I became pretty good at it. However, I could never feel fulfilled as it was all efforts to fix my shattered confidence through pleasing her, which was impossible to do because she could no longer affirm me.

I emotionally refused to take any of her affirmation of me sexually because I went so many years believing I was this great lover for her, while I was inadequate to the degree she sought upgrades.

Sex became nothing but a performance-based void for me. I would achieve a moment of gratification if I thought I did good. Then, the very next time, I was back to square one of feeling pressure, anxiety, and inadequacy. I was loading myself up with oral and injectable medications to get an erection and battling the severe performance anxiety that was consuming me.

Sex was terrifying, and BDSM triggered me to a place of anguish.

After some time, I tried to tell her I couldn't do the BDSM because of the mental pain it caused. Shortly after agreeing to stop, she started selfishly complaining that it was her preferred experience and that she was being deprived without it.

This, of course, triggered my insecurities and thoughts of her seeking it elsewhere. So, I started it again—pleasing her while sending myself deeper into a state of traumatic depression.

The medications I was using to get an erection—mainly the injections—were very painful to use and unpredictable, as I truly had no control over my erection going down. It also had the potential long-term side effects of creating scar tissue in the penis, which could make things worse. So, I was putting myself in mental and physical harm, trying to maintain this relationship.

I know what you're asking yourself. Why do it? Why not leave? Ironically, these are questions I've posed in a dismissive way to friends in abusive relationships or other traumatic circumstances.

This woman's actions and reasoning for cheating on me, combined with my preexisting trauma, had delivered me to a place of telling myself, "I have to hold on to her because who else will want me? Who is going to accept this broken man with a broken dick? What can I offer that's sustainable?"

So, not only could I not leave her, but I had to do everything I could to please her because it was my only hope. You start selling yourself on this shitty premise. It's a place of weakness and low self-worth I wouldn't wish on my worst enemy. The idea of going back into the world and finding a companion, with my inability to get an erection, was just something I could not consider. At least I knew she loved me.

She cared for me, and she expressed she wanted us to be together. That expression, along with my fear, compelled me into forgiving something that was unforgivable and caused constant torment.

Losing my ability to get an erection happened simultaneously with the betrayal trauma. My dick took precedence. All my focus was on correcting the erection issue, and my emotional pain took a back seat. I blocked it out because my entire self-worth depended on fixing my inadequacy as a lover.

So, emotional healing was out of the question. I found myself in a never-ending state of deep trauma as I continued to try to solve an emotional issue with a physical remedy.

This cycle of trying to fix my erection to ultimately fix everything else led, eventually, to getting an implant. It was the only ironclad way I could correct my erection issue with 100% certainty. Remove the anxiety, pressure, and insecurity that caused me to lose all function from being betrayed. Now that I could remove that physical trauma, emotional trauma was a non-issue. It gave me back the belief that I could find a woman for me, and I finally walked away from the therapist.

It wasn't easy. I believe we trauma-bonded in some way. I have made peace with the situation, and I am trying to find a place to understand that she, too, was broken and that the pain she caused me wasn't personal. It was just a byproduct of her maladaptive behavior. (she's currently still married and moved with her family out of state)

I still love and care for her and ultimately wish her all the best. It was the toughest period of my life, but now, because of the implant, I'm at least physically healed.

Now I can finally work on my heart because my dick is a formidable force to be reckoned with. This is how crazy life is—my woman completely shredded my life to pieces by going out and buying dick, which then motivated me to buy a dick for myself.

It ended up being the best thing ever to happen to me. Talk about when life gives you lemons… make lemonade! Hold my fucking beer 'cause I took that to a whole other level!

My Shitty Truth

Now that you heard my shitty story and the oh woe is me tale of a lifelong womanizing stripper that got his heart and dick broke in a grimy ass way, now that the smoke is clear, and I'm done crying, let's just be blatantly truthful about it. I was just at a weak, insecure, low-confidence place in my life when I met this woman.

She found a way to build me back up and give me what I needed most: my masculinity and my value. My place in life of not living up to the standard that would make me feel financially formidable, along with my iffy erection, had me in a mindset of I didn't even deserve an amazing woman.

So, when she came in the picture and made me feel that not only did I deserve an amazing woman, but she was grateful for the opportunity to have me, over time, it glued all my broken pieces together.

So, obviously when the truth came to light of her indiscretions, those freshly glued pieces were hit with a sledgehammer, and now I'm broken into thousands of pieces. Although I did eventually love her, her sole purpose as a woman in my life was to make me feel better about myself.

It was her entire value. The truth is, she was definitely cute and had a nice body... notice like my other stories I didn't rave about how gorgeous/fine she was, etc. The truth is, she was below my standard. Someone I was settling for in my mind.

So, to be in a place where you believe you are settling and going below your standards, you believe no way this person is going to fuck up on me. I'm like hitting the lottery for her! I could take my young, beautiful single girls from my past who cheated and hurt me for an NBA player.

As great as I thought I was, in my mind, that was an upgrade and made sense. But for my average old married chick to cheat and hurt me with a hired male prostitute was unbearable to my ego. I guess she left my dirty dick for a dirtier one... and as much as she tried to apologize and make it right (which she did for years), I could never move past it because it was never about LOVE.

It was always about my ego and confidence that she could no longer affirm... and without that, I could never truly value her. Fun fact: I've been bitching and moaning about this woman hiring a male prostitute and ironically the reason I met her was she hired ME TO FUCK HER! Clearly hiring dick is only acceptable if it's mine. Hypocrisy at its finest! So, I shouldn't had been surprised at all, but delusion and denial can run deep as fuck when you think you are the "special one" in someone's life.

Now, for the men who have lost their confidence and ego, who have true loving, caring, supportive women to put them back together, cherish her, and I applaud you. In my case, I had someone's wife who, in hindsight, should have never been in that position with me.

It was and always should have been my responsibility to fix within me what was broken: my mental state, my confidence, my broken heart, my finances, and definitely my dick. But it was easy for me to give up on doing the work.

Put responsibility in someone else's hands and then blame them when it goes bad like it's all their fault. I was a broken person relying on a broken person to fix me. Not exactly a recipe for success.

So, like we are supposed to do as men, I'm taking back my accountability. Being fully responsible for my happiness and peace of mind.

The Shitty Point

I share my sad tale of heartbreak because all of us men have a couple of these horror stories that have derailed our lives for a period of time. It's part of life and, honestly, essential to being a man. It builds us up in a way.

But as older men, especially those struggling with ED, the same experience that helped build us can completely break us. Just like I was broken and in denial that it was impacting my life far more significantly than I was aware of.

So many of us are sitting in the same denial. How many times have you heard stories of men in long-term relationships living with their spouses, sleeping in separate rooms? Years have passed and no sex. He's barely respected, belittled, and unappreciated. You can clearly see he has changed and is nothing like the guy he used to be.

If it's not us personally, we all have a friend or have at least heard of someone in this situation. Why does this happen? From the outside looking in, it's easy to say just leave. But the truth is, in many of these situations, the man is broken and has lost confidence in his ability to find a better partner.

So, a shitty relationship with a woman is better than no woman at all. So you just grin and bear it. But why? Why did you lose confidence in fixing your relationship or finding better? I guarantee you it has something to do with sexual confidence.

Look at my situation. The woman that I was dealing with had me and her husband. We were both exceptional earners, so confidence didn't waver there, but what we also had in common were sexual issues that killed our confidence.

So, we both hung on to her even with a history of betraying us at points in our relationships. But she was someone that had already stuck with us through our ED, so like the men I'm referring to, we just hung on to the terrible situation.

Money, material success—nothing could help me break away from that bad situation until I confidently corrected my sexual issue. So, if you or someone you know is currently living their shitty story, just functioning in their love life/ relationship in a shell of what it should be, being proactive and fixing your issues is your only chance to get back on track.

Please, brothers... I was there. It feels hopeless, but don't let your life die on that hill. Fight for your life; you know you deserve better. I knew I did, and the first place I started was with my sexual potency.

Don't Give Up On Your Sexual Potency

I gave up on my sexual potency and masculinity at one point, and my desperation at that time wasn't pretty. I was depressed, anxious, and thought I'd never experience intimacy and pleasure with a woman again, and the worst part of it was I was in complete denial.

Now, please understand that my issue did not make me incapable of sex. I could still get an erection and have a pleasurable experience. The depression was about the physical and mental process I went through to be capable of sex. When you are so consumed mentally with the process of sex, it becomes more of a chore than pleasure.

80

I had all but given up on carefree, enjoyable, fun sex like when I was younger. I was certain those days were over. But I was so very fucking WRONG. I didn't realize that I still had a whole lifetime of amazing sex ahead of me.

I am here to tell you not to give up on your sexual potency and pleasure, no matter what kinds of insane Reddit threads you've already read at 2 am, weird dick-enhancing mushrooms you've ordered, witchcraft remedies you've already tried, and doomsday thoughts you've had about your dick or the shitty story you went through.

If you don't make a conscious decision to make a change, you could find yourself turning a blind eye to survival.

CHAPTER FOUR

Turning a Blind Eye: The Crazy Things We Do to Avoid Facing Our Erectile Dysfunction

So yeah, you know this: erectile dysfunction can make us feel fucking terrible about ourselves, and it shows up all over our lives—most clearly in our relationships. We might feel guilty that we can no longer perform for our partners—one of the important ways that we feel good about ourselves in relationships.

For better or worse, a man's sexual performance is directly connected to feeling powerful and validated. When these feelings aren't regularly affirmed, it can create a void within us and around us. This void becomes a wall that may have a domino effect, deteriorating our relationships. Once this void is created, many relationships do not survive, and if they do survive, they live on in a diminished, weakened state. No one is feeling love or intimacy or having fun because everyone is anxious and sad.

ED also causes friction in relationships that show up in other areas that are not obvious. Our partners become frustrated, and feelings of failure, rejection, shame, and anxiety begin to swirl around both us and them. If we don't have an existing practice of healthy communication that we've worked on, it's hard to search openly for resolutions together. At some point, we may realize that sex is just not happening, and over time, we might become accustomed to that reality, silently suffering, but not actively working on it with our partners.

When there is no sex, emotional intimacy often suffers as well, and we might end up feeling disconnected, with resentment and insecurity getting in between ourselves and our partner. The sense of not feeling desired compounds all of this, creating endless escalating negative effects. This is how erectile dysfunction can become a passive wedge that slowly divides and conquers what was once a solid relationship. Petty spats can become massive disagreements. Where an argument that used to last between a day turns into a week, then two weeks, then three weeks. You get the picture? Culture tells us it's a man's job to fix these little spats—to reach for our partners in a healing, loving way. In better times, before our ED, these might be moments of intimacy that both partners look forward to. Sexual desire is a clear motivation to make peace with your partner because it's pretty clear that if she's upset, you most likely ain't getting none. But if you are suffering from ED, that motivation is void, which is a big part of resolving conflicts. Makeup sex is a thing! This can be a very important place for maintaining harmony, but even makeup sex can be missed out on when we're avoiding the reality of our erectile dysfunction.

ED may subconsciously hinder any effort to make our women happy and thwart our attempts to repair situations that weren't a big deal earlier in the relationship. Where we would reach out in an attempt at intimacy, now we may turn back inward, afraid to even put a hand on her back because that could lead to something that will cause us more anxiety.

So now, intimacy is no longer wonderful, shared moments with our lover. Intimacy itself is a performance issue and is something that creates uncomfortable pressure, activating our nervous system instead of relaxing us. To avoid it, we may create an excuse. We might avoid accountability. No man wants to look his woman in the eye and say, "I'm avoiding intimacy because I'm scared of my own anxiety," or "I'm not able to perform, and it scares me." Instead, we might hide behind a mountain of excuses to avoid disappointing our partner.

The truth is, this is the point where we should be stepping up, not backing down, but if you don't have an answer, how do you step up? Who is in a hurry to do something that makes them uncomfortable? As tough as we're supposed to be, we are deeply vulnerable, and this is not a comfortable place for most men.

All of this insecurity, hiding, and subconscious avoidance causes a lot of pain, but what's the end result? Very often, it's old-fashioned cheating—on both parts. A woman may seek intimacy with a man who makes her feel desired and can show up for sex. We may seek sex with someone who doesn't push our intimacy buttons, so it's just plain old fucking with no expectations.

As a male stripper, I used to take advantage of the classic scenario of women in failing relationships. Like, A LOT. I cannot tell you how many women I've come across in sexless marriages. I know this happens for various reasons, but I also know that a lot of it is a direct result of erectile dysfunction, because I've talked to both the men who've experienced it and talked to (and fucked!) the women on the other side of it.

When sexual performance begins to fail and chemistry begins to evaporate, partners give up on trying to have sex with each other, filling those voids outside of the relationship.

Ironically, men with ED are *more likely to cheat.* I know that sounds confusing, and you might be wondering: If you can't perform at home, why would you go out and seek to fail elsewhere? Imagine how devastated women are when they find out their spouse, the guy with performance issues who gave up on sex with her, is now fucking around. She's going to be both furious and sad, overflowing with insecurity and shame.

It's just another attempt to avoid the pressure of sexual decline. When a relationship starts, our sexual performance is top-notch, and from there, we build connection, confidence, and security with a partner. We may set a sexual standard for ourselves that we take for granted.

If you're out cheating with a casual connection, there's less of a need to perform and impress. This lower standard might make you feel more comfortable with the random chick than you do in your actual relationship.

Cuckolding is a term used to describe situations where a man gives consent for his partner to sleep with other men (and usually wants to watch) is a lot more common than you may think. What people don't realize is that this happens a lot when men have ED—since they can't perform and they want their partner to be satisfied, they put another man in charge of that business. Now, I hold no judgment against anybody and their kinks. I understand some men get off by watching their women deal with other men, and that's a sexual fantasy of theirs… to each his own.

But getting personal, I am an only child, and I am extremely possessive and territorial. The idea of any man interacting with my woman sexually is an absolute no-no. I used to hear about cuckolding and think: *hell to the motherfucking no. I would never.* This is how I am to the core.

But when I went through a period where I couldn't perform sexually for the first time in my life, not only did cuckolding make sense, but I convinced myself it was what I needed to do. I started thinking of the terms, parameters, and details I could live with. My partner had an extremely high libido, was very sexual, and wanted to fuck frequently. To make matters worse, my sexual issues were directly connected to her cheating on me and saying my diminished performance and lack of variety were the factors that led her astray. This blow to my confidence left me a shell of myself as a lover.

So now, even though I'm the guy that would break up with my girl for just dancing with some dude in the club, I'm thinking about how to get my partner a new partner, just to keep her satisfied. I was ready to turn a blind eye and let her seek sex from other men with my consent, which went against every fiber of my being.

As a male stripper, this is a very standard thing to come across—a couple has already gone years in a "don't see, don't care" scenario where they operate with impunity. These couples are together, and they are in a sexless relationship where the woman is doing her thing while her man turns a blind eye. As long as he doesn't know about it, she can do what she wants, as long as she doesn't embarrass him or the family or deal with any man in their circle of friends and no one finds out about it. These rules are bent and accepted by men who probably would never, ever consider a dynamic like this, but many of them are only doing it because of impaired sexual performance.

The first time a guy hired me to sleep with his wife, ironically, I had already slept with his wife.

A couple of years earlier, I met his wife while doing a show in St. Martin in the Caribbean. She was there vacationing, and I had sex with her. (I had no recollection of this happening. I'm not saying it didn't, but my level of hoeness at the time was $2 hooker level). She returned home and told her husband about how amazing the sex was with me. A few years later, I did a show in Toronto, Canada, where they lived. Her husband sought me out at the show, pulled me to the side, and said, "I want to hire you for my wife. She had an experience with you. She said it was the best of her life. I want that to happen again."

At this point, I had not been exposed to any cuckolding scenarios, so I was *confused as fuck*. Although I was dealing with the start of my ED issues, I had no idea why someone would be okay with me sleeping with his wife… and yet hire me to sleep with her again. But I wasn't going to turn it down. The fact that she said I was the best ever was high-octane ego fuel, so who was I to deprive her of another moment of stud ecstasy? His wife was super sexy, fit, attractive, and looked to be in her late thirties. Plus, to sweeten the deal, he offered me $500! So you mean I get to smash this sexy lady's buns *and* get paid for it? No-brainer—count me in!

This guy looked maybe ten years older than me, but still young. I mean, he probably was in his early to mid-40s, clearly successful and good-looking. Not at all the type of guy you would think hires a guy to bang his wife. I was truly stuck with the thought, *Why the hell would he want to hire me for this?*

I was really naïve about it. No way in hell would I have let my wife do it or even consider it! But it is what it is, and if he wanted it done, then it was going down! So we agreed, and he was bringing her to my hotel later. His only stipulation was condoms, and he needed to be in the room to make sure she was okay. Now, him needing-to-be-in-the-room part kind of weirded me out. So you want to watch me bang your wife? I immediately started to worry, thinking, *I'm going to be smashing and this dude is going to creep up from behind and try to put his thumb in my butt!* I was like, "Bro, what do you mean you want to be there?" He assured me he was a straight man, and there would be no funny business. He said that being there was for his wife to be comfortable, as it had been some years since she and I had connected. I wasn't really comfortable with his reasoning, but $500 to fuck a hot chick is $500. So, it was a go.

I rushed back to the hotel and started getting ready. Like any self-respecting guy with integrity and professionalism, I immediately told my friends! "Dude, this guy's bringing his hot wife by for me to smash her for five hundred fucking dollars! Y'all got to get the fuck out!" I was with my boys, Gee and Dig. They had so many questions of what, where, when, and how. As I filled them in on the details, my friends were like, "No fucking way! You the man!" which I completely agreed. "*Yes!* I am the man. This is what happens when you sling high-quality dick across the globe." I just continued to bask in all my glory, telling my friends that one day they may be lucky enough to sling dick like me, the super stud extraordinaire!

With all the talking and gloating, time flew, and the couple had arrived. Honestly, I did this purposely because I wanted Gee and Dig to see how hot the wife was, which would just give me more street cred with my boys. Legendary status, here I come!

The husband knocked on the door, and I let them in. The wife was in a short mini skirt, looking too good to be true. Gee's and Dig's mouths dropped as she was actually hotter than I described. I immediately assured the couple, "Hey, don't worry. These guys are about to leave," and I give my boys the *time-to-go* look.

As I cleared space for their exit, the husband said, "Wait," whispered to his wife briefly and then said, "Why don't you guys stick around and hang with us, too?"

I went straight Arnold from *Different Strokes*. "Whatchu talkin' 'bout, Willis! What do you mean?"

My boys immediately said, "Fuck yeah, we'll hang!"

In my mind, I'm like, *Fuck no! I'm an only child. I don't share.* This was my stud muffin moment, but as you know, I couldn't voice this as I would be hating and breaking rules 3-17 of the universal guy code(it ain't no fun if the homies can't have none), so I played it cool.

The husband told his wife to go to the bathroom to freshen up, and then he pulled us to the side to talk. "Look, fellas. I'm sure you know why we are here, and I want the three of you to show my wife the time of her life! Don't worry about me. Anything goes! Tear her to pieces! Is $500 each good?"

he said to Gee and Dig. They didn't even verbally respond. They just looked at each other in this devious way, stuck their hands out, and took the cash.

So now it was the three of us for his wife and I was like, *What the fuck!* But you know what? I got paid. I wasn't giving this money back, so the show must go on.

His wife came out of the bathroom. The husband gave her the "Go ahead, honey, have fun," and sat down on a chair on the other side of the room.

Now I was the reason why she was there, so I led her to the bed and began my stud muffin techniques. I started kissing her neck. She started moaning. I started rubbing her sensually all over her body. I could tell she was really getting into it, and the moment was right. As I began really turning up the heat, things took a very sudden and unexpected turn.

Now Gee and Dig are two of my closest friends. I mean, you can even call us family. There may not be two guys I could say I know better, but let me tell you—what you know about your friends in typical daily life situations can be *extremely* different in sexual scenarios because these guys morphed into something fucking different! That devious look they gave each other earlier was now an actual energy. It felt like an exorcism was about to begin, and the demons were entering the room!

So, I continued making my moves on the wife and suddenly, Gee started saying some of the craziest, outlandish shit I've ever heard!

"Oh yeah, baby, I'm gonna shove this dick in your mouth so deep, I'm gonna feel your thoughts."

"Oooh yeah, baby. I want to rub my sweaty balls on the back of your neck while I shoot my jizz on your skull."

He went next-level pervert, like a satanic version of Quagmire from *Family Guy*. And to make it even worse, he was talking in this weird, loud, macho man, Randy Savage, the wrestler's voice! I was like, "Who the fuck is this guy?"

Dig wasn't loud and crazy like Gee, but he was a focus killer on a different level altogether. Now, Dig is a slight dude, to say the least. I'm talking five-foot-seven, maybe one hundred sixty pounds without a muscle on his body. The guy that makes no effort to work on his physique, but makes up for it by being a fly guy — always sharply dressed and has the gift of gab with the ladies. For context, think a young hip-hop version of Mr. Burns from *The Simpsons*. So Dig was honestly a guy I couldn't even begin to think about in a sexual situation because I was confused about how he got girls in the first place. So what I learned about Dig this day is forever imprinted in my brain. Dig got naked and, as I said, not a muscle in sight. But this dude had a whole hoagie! I'm talking a hero sandwich straight from Subway and not the six-inch, but the twelve-inch. To this day, I can't hear the Subway commercial jingle, "$5…$5…$5 foot loooong," without a visual of Dig. It's terrible!

Another thing I knew was that Gee and Dig had been friends since middle school, and growing up, it was common practice for them to tag team chicks sexually, and boy, did I underestimate their chemistry. My warmup of sensual kissing and touching quickly became a WWF steel cage royal rumble match as Dig and Gee put the smackdown/battle royale/royal rumble on this guy's wife, while the whole time Gee called play-by-play in his Randy Savage voice. It appeared they had a sexual version of all the top wrestling moves.

91

I saw a butt-naked camel clutch, Boston crab, DDT, figure 4 leg locks, the brain buster, the jack hammer, tombstone piledrivers, toehold step over face lock, head scissors, and most impressively, a leapfrog body guillotine. You name it, they did it.

They turned this woman into a piñata and used their dicks to knock the candy out of her. I was in awe. All this was out of my comfort zone, and I just tapped out. I couldn't even perform. Between Gee's Randy Savage perverted outburst, "Let me cum on your kneecaps," and Dig's whole wheat hoagie and the steel cage match happening on a queen-sized mattress. I was slightly traumatized, so an erection was out of the question. I ended up just having a conversation with the husband, as I'm looking at him sitting calmly through his wife gasping for air while being washboarded by sweaty balls.

So, I had to ask. "Bro, why are you doing this?"

"Listen, me and my wife have been together for a bunch of years. I love her dearly. At some point in our relationship, sexually, I just could not continue to perform. I know I can't satisfy her the way she wants. She's still a young woman, and she has her needs. If I say, 'Just go out there and find your sexual partner,' it's risky to me as I feel most women can't just have sex detached. So I don't wanna send her out there to fulfill her sexual needs and then she meets some guy that she's intimate with and develops attachments and feelings." He went on, "What if he starts saying, 'Be with me. Leave him. We can be together?' I can't risk that! I still love my wife. So the only way I can get her satisfied without the risk of losing her is by finding the guys myself. I'm there, I'm in control. I control the interactions. So this person doesn't try to steal my woman. I don't like it, but I gotta make the most of it because I love my wife, and I don't wanna lose her."

It was clear to me that if he could satisfy her, he wouldn't want this. He wasn't necessarily happy about it. It was something he was policing because he didn't want to get divorced and lose his money, assets, and his foundation—and most importantly, his great love. All of this was added to their marriage because of his inability to perform. I believe there's a lot of that. Essentially, he was just turning a blind eye...but not just to his wife. More importantly, to himself. He was defeated. He gave up, tapped out of the fight because of his own sexual inabilities. Now this guy was loaded. If I had the financial means to correct my ED issue, he certainly did. But he accepted his circumstances, most likely because he didn't want to face how he felt.

The moral of this particular story: don't turn a blind eye. Stay in the fight. Fix your ED by any means necessary! Don't tap out. And if you haven't already, rise from the dead like the WWF legend THE UNDERTAKER and get back in the fight. You have to, because if you don't, there could be two guys like Gee and Dig putting a Battle Royale Tag Team Smackdown on your lady! Macho man voice included!

CHAPTER FIVE

Dysfunction Junction: Everything That Can Go Wrong
Physically With Your Cock and Ways to
Fix It (And Ways Not to Fix It)

So yeah—we've established again and again that poor mental health is the biggest detriment to your dick. Nine times out of ten, your mind is what's the matter with your cock, and with love, attention, communication, understanding, and therapy—you can fix it. Yes, sometimes it's about the body, and we have to rule out medical issues before we deal with what's in our heads. (More on that later.)

But shit, people hate to deal with their feelings, so they LOVE to turn to substances first. And the big problem with that is that most of the things people used to fix dick problems are going to give you…worse dick problems.

Let's take weed. We love weed. I have nothing against weed, but man, weed knows how to fuck up an erection fast. Some people claim that weed makes them horny, and that may be true, so some dudes like to smoke before sex. But weed can quickly turn your erection soft —it is notorious for killing an erection mid-fuck. This also goes for weed gummies. They relax you… but a bit too much.

Next up on the downward dick spiral is alcohol. Too much of it can also cause erectile dysfunction, though temporarily. If you're an alcoholic, nine out of ten times, you can't get your dick up. Have you ever had too much to drink one night, and the next day you were drinking glasses of water like a fish? Alcohol—for example, beer—is a diuretic that causes frequent urination and can result in dehydration, which decreases the volume of blood in the body and also decreases blood flow to the penis, making it more difficult to get an erection.

So, in layman's terms, when you're with a hot woman and you're ready to get busy, and you've been boozing, your brain tells your dick to do one thing, but the liquor is holding your dick captive. No erection for you.

Lesbian By Choice

One of the perks of being the top male stripper was that I got to travel all over the world for work. One weekend, I lucked up and got a show at the Atlantis in the Bahamas. The woman who hired me was… just wow! She was gorgeous. Her name was Janet, a super-sexy, tall blonde, bisexual white girl from Kansas who was wild as hell. Party girl to the 10th power… think young Jessica Simpson looks with prime Dennis Rodman's personality.

She actually lived in Miami, and the hotel flew her to the Bahamas every single weekend to entertain high rollers. It was her job to entertain them and provide them with whatever they wanted: parties, hookers, drugs, you name it. Her sole purpose was to keep them entertained, which led to them spending more money in the hotel/casino, and Janet was the best at this! One of her clients was having their high-profile wedding, and Janet flew me in to perform at the bachelorette party. "Nice! Paid vacation in the Bahamas," I can't wait.

Unfortunately, I flew in, and as soon as I landed, I got

the bad news that the bachelorette party had canceled me! The groom got wind of me being hired and was not going to let me put my balls on his bride's forehead in exchange for monetary gain. Disappointing, but I must say... smart guy!

Janet picked me up from the airport, apologized, then suggested, "Hey, you're already here; stay and hang out. Maybe I can get you some other gigs. You can stay in my room with me." Now, getting me some other gigs sounded cool and was a nice gesture, but let's keep it real... we know what "stay in my room with me" means. Janet wanted my not-so-Jamaican beef in her patty... Bumbaclot.

My prediction was accurate, and we were fucking ALL weekend long. And it was off the chain! The best combo of great sex and toxic dysfunction. Janet was one of those women that can appear like the coolest, sweetest, awesome woman all day long, aka Jessica Simpson, then four shots of tequila, a half a joint, and a mysterious pill or line of cocaine from a random stranger, and here comes this muthafucking Dennis Rodman.

She's cussing out people, passed out in the corner, urinating in inappropriate places, and I'm just along for the ride trying to hold her together. As crazy as this sounds, and I have no idea why at times we are sucked in on these people that are total chaos, but I truly couldn't get enough of her! Now this relationship with Janet took place while I was still heavy in my stud muffin era.

So I was definitely proving the theory of "once you go black, you never go back," because Janet was SPRUNG! She was literally addicted to sex, and she made that abundantly clear by continuously flying me to see her in the Bahamas for the next eight weekends straight.

Since she worked at the hotel, she would get a comp room that I could just stay in with her. It was a free, weekly vacation for me, amazing sex, and something crazy was guaranteed to happen, so why not? Basically, she had shifts where she would be busy entertaining the high rollers, whether in the casino, club, or cabanas. When her shift was over, she and I would hang out. It was two months straight of paradise that, get a load of this… was going to get extremely better.

So, Janet's birthday rolls around, and she wanted to celebrate in the Bahamas, but this time the plan was to celebrate her birthday at the Atlantis, along with two of her close girlfriends: Cookie, her best friend from Detroit, who was this big booty ratchet stripper girl (another fine ass Megan Thee Stallion/Cardi B vibes), and Ciarra, a private wealth manager from Mumbai, who was this tall, classy, sophisticated, gorgeous, curly-headed Indian girl (think dark-haired Zendaya).

Both were, at some point, Janet's lovers, and for her birthday, she wanted the four of us to get our freak on. Now, I know me and three beautiful women already sound amazing, but hold my beer, it gets much better!

So we all fly in on a Friday evening to the Bahamas, and we are all staying in a suite for the weekend. The plan is we are going to have dinner and then hit the nightclub located in the casino, then, of course, back to the room for the freak off. We get to the club, and I'm going big baller style, so I buy us a prime VIP section in the middle of the dance floor with four bottles of the best alcohol! Let the party begin.

Now, I didn't know or remember anyone in this club aside from the girls I was with, but I assure you, everyone in there remembers me because I was the poster boy for the saying, "THIS GUY IS THE FUCKING MAN." I'm literally with the three hottest girls in the club, and they are all over me, all over each other, making out. Security had to come by multiple times and reluctantly tell me, "Dude, it's too crazy over here. You have to tone it down," while simultaneously fist-bumping and professing I'm their idol.

In the midst of the chaos, Janet picked up this smoking hot European model (think young Bridgette Neilsen), and they started making out, and Ciarra picked up a Hispanic mother and daughter duo. The mother was around forty and understandably not as hot as the other girls, but definitely fuckable. The daughter, on the other hand, was around twenty-one and sexy (think low-budget Kris and Kylie Jenner)! They were on a family vacation and decided to come with us back to the room. So now I'm about to have a United Nations-style orgy! Me and six fucking women!

We all get back to our hotel room, and it immediately goes crazy. Janet pulls the European model to the king-size bed, and they start undressing and making out. The Hispanic mother sat on the couch alone and just watched while Ciarra and her daughter started to make out. I'm watching this unfold, and it doesn't seem real. It's like everything is happening in slow motion on silent, and all I hear is the hook of this Nas rap song, "Whose world is this? It's Sharay's, it's Sharay's, it's Sharay's."

Suddenly, Cookie just grabbed me, and it was clear she wanted it. She was roommates with Janet, so she'd been hearing for months about the filet mignon quality penis I was serving her BFF.

The couch and bed were occupied, so Cookie just pulled me to the front door of the room and just bent over and pulled her skirt up, "Gimme that dick!" OMG, this has to be awesome, right? Wrong. Horribly wrong. I'd been drinking so much; I could not get my shit fully hard. The dreaded half boner. It's like my dick woke up, got dressed for work, walked to the front door, opened it, and said, "Fuck it, I'm calling out today," and went back to bed. With those feeble half boners, all you can do is try to squeeze your dick at the base and smash it in her vagina with the hopes you get enough friction to eventually get hard. Now, this technique has a high failure rate sober, so drunk AND A CONDOM is pretty much hopeless. But shit, I'm gonna try.

So, I was behind Cookie with the death grip at the base of my dick trying to penetrate her vajayjay, and it was the equivalent of trying to slice your steak with a spoon. After about 3 or 4 minutes of appearing like I couldn't find the hole, Cookie, in true Detroit ratchet chic fashion, turned to me and said, "What the fuck's wrong with yo dick, nigga?" Um…everything after those tender words of encouragement. Any chance of us fucking after that was dead! I just blamed it on the alcohol, and she turned around, sat on the floor, and started scrolling on her phone with a look of disgust/disappointment.

I just avoided any eye contact and scurried across the room to Ciarra. The night was young, so I was on to the next. Ciarra and I got a little bit of something going as she started to give me head, which popped my dick up immediately, but I must give her a resounding thumbs up to her multitasking talent level because while giving me head, she was simultaneously fingering the Hispanic daughter. I must say, at the time, I thought I was skilled at pleasing a woman with my fingers, but Ciarra took this shit to another level. It was like she was playing a sexual version of rock, paper, scissors in fast forward on this young woman's vagina, and obviously, it was super effective because this poor girl was howling like an American werewolf in London. It literally was loud, crazy sounds that I never heard or imagined being associated with sex. The only way I can describe it is to imagine a deaf person drunk in a bar loudly singing "Sweet Home Alabama."

Between my confusion and feelings of inadequacy of the rock, paper, scissors technique I clearly didn't have in my toolbox and the Hispanic daughter's Helen Keller howls, my dick's not showing up here. I had to keep it moving.

The next stop was over to Janet and the European model, which was a sight. As I said earlier, Janet was a young Jessica Simpson, and the European model was giving young Bridgette Neilsen, so the level of sexy was through the roof. They were so into each other in this soft, sensual way, as if no one else was in the room but them. Like one of those cable TV soft porn sex scenes on Cinemax, I could hear the cheesy background music in my head. So I had to be pretty smooth with this, as it was pretty clear all night that the model was primarily into Janet. "Got to play this just right." Janet and the EM are kind of in a facing cuddle position, making out and rubbing each other's bodies. So, I lay on the bed behind Janet like I was spooning her and started rubbing her back and lightly kissing her neck.

She then grabbed my hand and pulled it around her, putting it on her tits while at the same time EM reached forward and started rubbing my arm. "YESSSS, things are trending in the right direction." Now I didn't have a serviceable boner yet, but damn it, I was on the right track. As the moment started to progress and everything appeared to be going perfectly, Janet's split personality/alter Dennis Rodman ego just showed, and she popped up on the bed between me and EM and just randomly yelled, "CIARRA, could you shut that bitch up?" Like WTF, it's my fucking birthday. This is some bullshit.

Her being annoyed at the Helen Keller howls set her off, and she proceeded to cuss the whole room out. But everyone was drunk/high and barely acknowledging her, so she jumped out of bed and sat by herself at a nearby table, lit a blunt, and started blasting super loud on her Bluetooth speaker "STUNTING LIKE MY DADDY" by Lil Wayne. The European model ran over to console her, and I tried to follow suit, but I was swiftly rejected with "WHY DON'T YOU GO BACK TO COOKIE, since she obviously was more important than me."

Cookie heard her and rushed over and said, "Nah, bitch… nobody wants your fucking man. You playing yourself," as they gathered in further discussion in the corner by the table, arguing and passing the blunt at the same time. I just stood there in silence, like, *Please can I just catch a break?* The universe heard my thoughts, and Ciarra came and grabbed me. "Don't worry about Janet; she does this all the time. She won't even remember this in the morning. I need you."

"You need me?" I said to myself, thinking, *Yes! Another chance…* So I thought, but it wasn't what I expected. Ciarra then proceeded to tell me she was trying to have a good time

101

with the daughter, but she was uncomfortable with her mom there. So she asked if I could please occupy the mom; she was into me.

Now, being a strict follower of the universal guy code, my wingman instincts kick in, and most importantly, my "think with your dick" reasoning sold me on the idea that if I do this favor for Ciarra, I'll earn some brownie points to possibly fuck her later. I went over and sat next to the mom, and Ciarra immediately took the daughter out on the balcony.

So, I was on the couch trying to set it off with Mom, but Ciarra clearly restarted her rock, paper, scissors fingering routine, and Lil Miss Teen Wolf started that Helen Keller howl again ("Sweet Home Alabama" cued) "SMAMMEEET OOOOME ARRRRMAARAMA!" Mind you, this was on the balcony at 4:00 a.m., and I was sure all of Paradise Island could hear her now. JEEZ… So now, yet again, I was getting distracted, which for me spelled D-I-C-K-retracted. I had to do something!

Then my light bulb went off! In a situation like this, where the moment is too chaotic to get a boner, your best bet is some privacy. So I pulled the mom into the bathroom and shut the door. Yes! Finally, this may work! I picked her up on the sink, and it was crystal clear she was ready to fuck, but I needed a place of confidence. So I did what any upstanding dude would do—I ate pussy. Num num num num num num num num. I just buried my head deep between the HM's legs to really get into the zone. So much so that her thighs smashed on the side of my ears, and I got one of those noise-canceling studio headphone effects as if I had buried my head underwater.

This moment of calm during the storm was the perfect time to get my anxiety down and get back into the game. I escaped to this meditative state where all sound is drowned out to just the faint, distant background moans of HM while I'm nun-chuck-tonguing her vajayjay. In an effort to take advantage of this solemn moment, I decided to give myself some spiritual, positive, encouraging self-talk to put my mind in the right place. "PLEASE, please, God. Don't do this to me, pleeeese. It's six bitches in here. I'm one of your children. Let my dick resurrect from the dead like that other dude you helped out. I promise to turn my life around. Just please!"

So, in the tranquil peace of the thigh lock and my desperate Dick Kumbaya, my ol' "eat her pussy until your anxiety goes down" trick was starting to work, and the blood was starting to circulate in my groin area. My dick was starting to grow. It was moving at the pace of my eighty-year-old grandma trying to walk up a flight of stairs, but eventually, she gets to the top, and so will I! Has God answered my prayers? Maybe. It actually makes sense. Janet is an Aries, so we were in April, which was around Easter. Could this be? My dick's EASTER? The Res-ERECTION! My mind and thoughts started to return to the present moment, and it's perfect timing as in the background I hear the Hispanic mom let out a muffled "Ayyy yai yaiiiiiii" as Bruce Lick has entered the dragon once again, another conquered coochie to climax!

I pop my head from between her legs with confidence. My boner's back, and he's ready to party. I reach in my pocket for a condom as time is of the essence, as I mentioned

103

earlier. Hard-to-achieve erections melt like butter on a grill outside a hole. As I tear the condom packet simultaneously, I'm returning from the quiet of the thigh lock, and normal sound is now returning. As I regain my senses, the first thing I hear outside the bathroom door is Cookie going full Rodman. "Fuck ya'll and this bitch-ass hotel!" Then shortly after, hotel security yells, "EVERYBODY OUT NOW!"

Apparently, a combination of Teen Wolf getting rock, paper, scissors fingered on the balcony, howling loud as a motherfucker, and Janet blasting her Miami gangster rap to set the mood prompted half the hotel to call and complain about us. Mom jumps off the sink, quickly pulls her dress down, and runs out of the bathroom, grabbing her daughter and rushing out of the room with Euro Model right on her heels. The Rodman twins, Janet and Cookie, are belligerently arguing with security. "You're all hating because you could never get a bitch like me!"

Ciarra quietly and calmly slips out of the room with her travel bag so smoothly you would have never thought she was with us, and within 15 minutes, we were all escorted off the premises. Obviously, it was not going to be my dick's Easter, and the Res-Erection was a fail. The moral of this story is: I was one guy, and I had six women to myself and got no pussy—zero, zilch. And I'm not saying the night would have been completely different, but I truly believed I would have taken down at least two if I was responsible with my alcohol consumption. So please, my brothers, be responsible with your drug and alcohol use, as you could easily end up like me: in a room full of hot bisexual girls and be a "lesbian by choice."

Eat It If You Can't Beat It!

Yes, as men, we can decide to identify as lesbians. Sounds crazy, I know, but hear me out. With erectile dysfunction, we give up on our penises and start to talk about how well we eat pussy. Yeah, this hearkens back to my Bruce Lick days from a couple of chapters ago. Us male lesbians find ourselves buying vibrators, dildos, and other sex toys to compensate for our lack of performance. Not only are we giving up on fucking, we're giving up on us. Instead of addressing our problem, we overcompensate by trying to skill ourselves in other ways. As you know, it's good to have skills! But not to make up for not being able to fuck properly.

Some men are okay with toys because they know they can't offer penetration at all. But the guy that has wavering penetration may be anti-dildo because the dildo symbolizes intimidation. The dildo is going to be hard, which is something he's not. Some guys who aren't even experiencing erectile dysfunction aren't keen on toys in the bedroom because of this intimidation. I know I wasn't. I once felt like I was going to give myself an aneurysm trying to eat the pussy of a woman that routinely used a powerful vibrator. It was not fun at all!

So yeah, I chose to be a lesbian in the Bahamas that night. After that fiasco, I also chose to reduce my alcohol intake.

- High blood pressure
- Heart disease
- Obesity
- High cholesterol
- Sleep disorders

- Parkinson's disease
- Alcoholism
- Low testosterone
- Steroid use

I'm not going to dig into all the other health issues because I'm not a doctor, and you should see your doctor if any of those are your problem. But I'm very familiar with steroid use, hormonal imbalance, and testosterone and how important it is—so let's drill down.

Low T has many causes, but one I want to emphasize here is the dangers of steroid use. People pretty much know that steroids are bad news, but mainly in terms of heart disease and liver damage. But most people don't realize the other reason it should be avoided: it causes a hormonal imbalance that can straight FUCK up your libido. Our sex drive is controlled by our testosterone levels, and when you take steroids, you shut off your own reproductive system. Your body is not going to continue naturally making testosterone, and all your other hormones go completely out of whack.

It's almost impossible to regulate these hormones when you're adding artificial stuff in, and you just end up on a roller coaster of hormonal imbalance that can be terrible for your dick. Now, this isn't a Nancy Reagan "just say no to drugs" campaign against steroids. If you know what you're doing, you should be able to navigate these waters. This is for the average mid-life crisis guy who wants to try something new to fast-track some gains and may not be clear that's also the fast-track to a life of lesbian sex… Bruce Lick style.

So many of us guys who take care of ourselves and get into weightlifting might experiment with this stuff and then inadvertently shut their systems down. Maybe you do this once or twice at an early age, and it's not a big deal; your body usually can recover and reset itself, and you'll be okay.

But when you start fooling around with this stuff on the regular, especially over the age of 30, what you're doing is speeding up the clock of your decline. Whereas a normal 30 or 35-year-old man should have testosterone levels in the 800-900 range, especially if he's not abusing alcohol and marijuana. Using steroids will drop your levels to 0, so when you stop taking it there is none in your system. Your body then tries to restart itself and even if you do PCT (post cycle therapy) to help the restart, you may only get your natural levels back to a 600.

Healthy testosterone can be anywhere from 300 to 1200, depending on the scale you're using, so every time you take steroids and they completely shut you down, you come back to lower and lower and lower baselines.

For example, in your mid-thirties, your testosterone is beginning a normal decline—you lose a little bit every year. If you didn't use steroids, your decline may begin at 1200, so you'll hold out a lot longer before you drop to numbers that can affect your performance. But the guy that used steroids—his decline may start at a baseline of 600 because he's already lost so much.

You may still function fine if your decline begins from 600, but you'll get to your demise much quicker than those descending from 1200. So one of my biggest issues was using testosterone over 30 and starting my decline early, which then became an issue down the line.

Another part of this, which may be the real secret behind why a lot of men go through testosterone issues or erection issues without knowing it, is all the new wave diets people have been on in the last few decades. I was trying to stay lean and cut, so I went on one of those "keto" diets. This is when you cut all your carbs and sugar and you keep yourself lean by reducing your calorie intake.

From an aesthetic standpoint, it worked great—I slimmed down and was totally cut. I followed this for years, mostly because I liked the look , but what they don't tell you about these diets is that they can easily put you in a starvation mode mistaken as "ketosis." When your body is in starvation mode, it starts to shut down certain systems and regulates your hormones differently.

In my case, being in starvation mode for a long period of time imbalanced my hormones. There is a hormone, SHBG—sex hormone binding globulin. When you keep your body in starvation mode, you can raise your SHBG, and this essentially binds to your free testosterone. This means the free testosterone that you need for your sex drive and healthy erections is not available for me to use. This basically crashed my libido, so I was in a confusing circumstance where my testosterone levels were high enough for me to function normally, but nothing was normal. My total testosterone was 650, but my free testosterone was at 3. Free testosterone should be somewhere between 20 and 50 at worst, and I was at 3.

So, this is all to say that I had to start taking TRT to try to elevate my testosterone levels to compensate for the free T that was binding to the SHBG. And TRT is a whole other can of worms. So just be really conscious and aware of your eating habits, and never allow yourself to be in starvation mode. Eat balanced meals, get all those nutrients, and avoid those extreme diets. That calorie deficit shit is bad news.

CHAPTER SIX

Stock Your Toolbox: All the Correctives For Your Cock

So, by now, you know that I have VERY advanced experience with erectile dysfunction, leading up to me doing the Holy Grail Corrective: an implant. But before I got there, I went through every single possible option trying to correct it on my own, including some very questionable shit! In this chapter, I'm going to run down the list of things I did and rabbit holes I fell down to give you a lay of the land and allow you to make your own decisions about what to bother with if you're not ready to pull out the big guns (an implant).

A big caveat: I'm not a medical professional; I know my shit, but I'm a fucking male stripper, dudes. So I have plenty of advice, but it's NOT medical advice, and you're going to have to make sure to get the good word from your doctor after you read this. Don't just run to some Canadian cheap drug site or local sex shop—although I know most of you have already! But for the legality of things, be careful with your dick (and your heart and the rest of your body).

Supplements

Like many of us, I got hit with ED the first time at a very young age and started trying to correct it through regular Vitamin Shoppe/GNC supplements. For a healthy person or a moderately healthy person, these vitamins can give you some sort of help, but in my opinion, it's very minimal. You'll get ginseng and horny goat weed, and somebody will tell you to take vitamin C, and then it'll be watermelon juice with lemon. Then, some sort of "testosterone-boosting" supplement will come along.

One of my buddies who took deer antler velvet and swore by it convinced me to try it. He was like, "Man, this deer antler velvet makes me hard as a rock!" and lo-and-behold, I took it and had a great erection the first time. Bottom line: I really think the majority of this stuff creates a major placebo effect. Yes, there is scientific proof that a healthier way of life can help with erections, of course. Eating right, drinking enough water, exercising, and getting good sleep—this is going to help with your OVERALL health, so of course it's also going to help with your dick health.

And sure, if you're struggling with ED, you can go the healthy supplement route and have some success. If you go this route and get positive results, I'm very happy for you, man! But if you are truly struggling and you're trying to GNC/Vitamin Shoppe your way to good health, let's just be honest: it's a long shot, and now you've been warned.

Pharmaceuticals: Viagra and Cialis

After trying all the various supplements, usually getting your hands on some sort of pill is the next level. These pills range from the top of the chain—Viagra and Cialis, which are prescription pharmaceuticals—all the way down to what's behind the counter at your local gas station, some god-knows-what's-in-it pill from China. That motherfucker could actually have some dangerous shit in it, like Fentanyl, so no matter how desperate you are, maybe don't do that. Okay, I'm lying. When you're desperate for an erection, you're taking it, and so did I.

These FDA-approved pharmaceutical drugs (Viagra and Cialis) are very effective, specifically in the sense of the science behind them. What they do is expand your blood vessels; expanding your blood vessels in your penis allows for more blood, which gives you a strong erection. It's pretty simple.

What you're not told is that if you're struggling with ED or if you have any form of performance anxiety, that often contradicts the biological effects of these particular pills. So if you pop a Viagra or Cialis, your blood vessels will initially expand, but if you have self-doubt, worry, or intrusive thoughts like "Will my dick get hard? Will these pills work? Will I be able to perform?" your body may release a hormone called cortisol. This motherfucking cortisol will actually *constrict* your blood vessels, the *exact opposite* of what these pills are supposed to do for you.

This is why you may have had an experience where taking pills from the pharmacy or even random pills, ones that happen to have the same prescription drugs in them as Viagra and Cialis do, got you an erection, and you kept it because you *believed in the pill*. But if you tried a pill, and the anxiety spiked your cortisol, you'll then believe it's the pill's fault, so you'll move on to another pill. See how this works?

I've probably tried 20 different pills. With all of them, at some point, I had success, but it wasn't until after the fact that I realized all these pills were just the same medications

111

in a different package! The difference between the times they worked and the times they failed had only one factor: my own confidence. Sometimes, I'd have a whole bottle of Viagra in my house, but I'd jump in my car and drive 30 minutes in traffic to some gas station, frantic because I got a hookup with a girl later, and I believed in the specific pill.

One time, I drove 20 miles to a sex shop in the West Village to get something called Trio Power Zen 2000. Now, they have the 1200, the 1500, but I *needed* the 2000, and I would ride down there, buy this pill, pop it, and lo-and-behold, I'd get the Erection of Life. This was only because I was confident as fuck, but when I really did my research to see what's in Trio Power 2000, I found it's the *same stuff* that was in the big bottle of Viagra that I had in my medicine cabinet at home. Dude, I could have just stayed home.

I made the damn trip because I'd failed before with the Viagra, and I believed I might have a different experience with the Trio Power Zen—I didn't *know* it was Viagra, so I gave myself my own mind fuck.

In other words, if you know the pills are effective and they're going to change your blood vessels, if your mind is in the right place and you're not freaking out, you will likely get results. But if you are already in a place of anxiety and dealing with a fear of failure, you need to understand that this is the problem and driving across town and ordering pills from India and China—it's not gonna correct the circumstance because this is a situation where it is seriously all in your head. So if you are currently jumping from pill to pill to the chew, to the Honey or whatever you're taking, it's not the stuff—it's in your head. True story: one of my best friends ordered a bag of powder online that was supposed to give you erections. It looked like a kilo of cocaine, and the stuff smelled like a teenage boy with bad hygiene feet. We coined it the Athlete's foot, and my boy used to religiously ingest this random stink foot powder for sex. Man, the things we do to make love.

The Bootleg Boy Toy

In the heart of my pill dependency, I had another pure opportunity that became my usual disaster because of my lack of effort to fix my ED. I got a random call on a Saturday night from a female wanting to hire me. She said, "It's my birthday, and I'm here with a few girlfriends. Are you available tonight?"

Now, I usually would give last-minute parties away, but when I heard the location was Trump Tower Central Park West, I knew it was someone with big bucks, so I was keeping this gig. After some scheduling back and forth, I quoted her $200; we confirmed 2:30 a.m., and I showed up with my dance bag, ready to put on a show. I knocked on the door, and it opened to literally the most beautiful woman I had ever seen in person. I mean, she was flawlessly stunning. She greeted me with this huge, inviting smile, and it was clear she was in a bathrobe with nothing underneath. I'm startled yet in awe of her as she led me into the living room area of the hotel suite. The room was dimly lit but empty. I was expecting a room full of girlfriends celebrating with her, but no one was there, and oddly, all the furniture was covered in white sheets. When I saw this, my mind immediately flashed to the movie *American Psycho*, where the killer covered all his furniture in plastic before he killed someone, so I had a momentary freakout. I regained my composure, then asked, "Where would you like me to do the show?"

She responded that she wasn't interested in my dancing, and my purpose for being there was that her husband had a voyeur fetish and enjoyed watching her in sexy scenes. She wanted us to sit across from each other while sensually covering ourselves with baby oil. The goal was to make it look hot and sexy as possible while her husband watched from a distant corner across the room. Most importantly, we were supposed to act like her husband was not there and not acknowledge his presence at all.

She asked me to just change into a towel, pointed to a chair for me to sit in, and handed me $800 cash. Now, I was completely blown away and creeped out at the same time. Yes, this woman was gorgeous, but I really felt uncomfortable with this voyeur husband looking from afar, but fuck it, I was here, and I was definitely not giving back the $800. Just in case things escalated to more than a body rub, I took a 20-milligram Cialis to be ready.

We sat across from each other to start the scene, and I must admit, it was super sexy. She had this huge bottle of baby oil that was sitting in a bowl of hot water to make it warm. Then she drenched her body in it, limb by limb, rubbing herself all over while biting her lips. She appeared to be fully in the moment, and her energy was pulling me in. I started to get turned on and took the bottle, doing the same—covering my body with oil and rubbing it all over myself.

We sat across from each other, but close enough that if we both sat forward, we were within reach. We soon

114

started to rub and caress each other's bodies, and there was an apparent buildup of desire. As I'm caught up in this moment, I can't help but see movement from the corner of my eye. The husband had entered the room, and although he was not close to us, I could clearly make out what was going on. Dude was butt naked with one of those Muslim head coverings that only revealed his eyes, so his face is completely covered.

He has a bottle of Astroglide in his hand while he is madly whacking his meat with the other hand. Like, you could hear the whacking from across the room: wock wocc whoc wocc whoc.

Before I continue, I would like to make it clear that I have nothing against gay people. I support any way of life that one chooses. I have very close gay friends, but I am not a gay or bisexual man.

So, to have another dude in the background, naked and beating off, was way out of my comfort zone. I couldn't help but worry if this guy would make a move on me, so I was definitely paranoid and overthinking. Now, I'm not supposed to acknowledge him, so he didn't say anything directly to me, but he was speaking in a low voice, giving subtle orders to his wife, sharing his wants and enjoyment.

A fun fact about me: after all my years in the club with the loud music, I can't hear for shit. This was making matters 10 times worse because in my discomfort at the moment, everything he said to his wife, my deaf, non-hearing interpretation, was all fucked up. An example would be if he said to his wife, "Baby, move over to the right," my non-hearing paranoid brain would hear, "Yum. I bet his asshole's tight." Or if he said, "I love that position you're in," my deaf interpretation would be, "I can't wait to penetrate him."

So between the crazy whacking noises and the bad hearing interpretations, I am creeped all the way out and my dick won't stay hard for shit, so ain't no fucking happening.

But even with the inconsistent erection, she says, "That was great, we can stop now," and hands me $1,200 more! This was in addition to the $800 when I showed up. That's $2,000 for about 45 minutes of baby oil play with a limp noodle. I was ecstatic! She then let me know she felt comfortable with me and wanted me to come back the next time they were in town. "Hell yeah, I'll be back!" But she also mentioned, "And next time I would like to go a little further." Ah shit, the pressure was on now; I got to get me and my dick on the same page. Couldn't sell out two times in a row.

The next time, same situation, and I popped another Cialis. But since it had already let me down, I traveled to a random sex shop and asked the clerk for the strongest thing he had. He gave me Dick Density Gold, said it was his best seller. I popped the pill and showed up, praying this pill worked better than Cialis. Now, I had no idea what was in this pill, but my first reaction was, oddly, I had to take a shit, but not a normal shit. Like an I-did-a-colon-cleanse-diarrhea-everything-needs-to-exit-your-anatomy shit. I was on the toilet for 30 minutes straight. A roll of toilet paper and a shower later, it was time to work, and we were back in the scene with the oil and naked bodies, but this time, I had the Erection of Life. Dick Density Gold came through big time.

The only thing was, along with the boner, came a splitting headache. My face turned flush red, and I'm pretty sure my heart was beating out of rhythm. I was trying to keep my composure during the scene, but I was on that thin line of getting paid to fuck the hottest woman of my life or calling 911 to stay alive.

Like any responsible adult male, I chose to fuck the hot chick for money! The couch-caressing oil action got so steamy that we decided to take the scene to the bedroom, and now it was really going down. I dived between her legs and started the Bruce-lick-tongue-kung-fu-enter-the-36-chambers style pussy eating, and she went crazy.

After about 10 minutes, it was batting practice, and I was Dick Density deep balling her like an MLB Hall of Famer. We were both loving the moment, and apparently the husband was too, as he appeared out of nowhere and slammed a stack of $100 bills on the bed, then said, "Oh yeah, I like this shit!" My asshole instantly clenched as my deaf ear heard him say, "He's about to get this dick." I began to feel the creeped-out energy and feared my boner was a goner. Luckily, he didn't say that, and my dick didn't go down either. This was the Erection of Life. Nothing could get it to go down. Nothing, nothing, nothing. No, I mean seriously, nothing! I literally could not get my dick to go down. My shit was petrified.

I lost all sensation. I couldn't feel shit; couldn't enjoy shit and couldn't cum for shit. My dick was just a dead log. After about an hour, she was begging me to cum, and I was using every focus technique I could think of to try to bust a nut, and it wasn't working. I was ready to call it quits, as she appeared satisfied, but it became clear that they weren't going to be happy unless I came also.

So eventually, I had to call timeout from the scene, and I jumped on Google for help with this Dick Density Gold erection. After some quick searches, I learned I needed to drink a glass of ice water to somehow help me ejaculate (I have no idea why, but I tried it, and it worked.)

So finally, I was able to blow my load, which she insisted I do all over her vagina! I shot her box up like she was the winning coach of the Super Bowl, and my dick was the bucket of Gatorade. She loved it and oddly I guess the husband did too, as this ending became the routine every time we got together, which at first was nice until over time I begin to suspect that after I blew my load, her hubby was helping her wipe up by licking her clean (overthinking, paranoid mind strikes again and I'm creeped out times 10).

So on and off for the next 3 years, I was the boy toy for this rich, powerful couple 5 to 6 times a year when they came to NYC. The problem was, because of the weird circumstances, I could only get an erection about 50% of the time to really sustain a good session. This started to put tremendous stress on me to perform, and I needed a solution. I couldn't lose this $2,000 a session.

My way of solving this problem? Just take more pills! Next time, the Dick Density Gold didn't work. So I tried the Platinum. Then I tried the Platinum with Cialis. Then the Platinum with Cialis and Viagra. Then a Platinum, a Gold, a Cialis, and a Viagra. You get where I'm going with this? I was completely overdosing on these pills, thinking the more I took, the better the result. Which is not how they work at all, and my erections remained inconsistent and completely unpredictable.

Eventually, my bootleg erection got me canned, and my boy toy gig was done. $2000 a night to fuck the most beautiful woman I'd ever seen, and I overdosed and over thought my way out of the opportunity. But in my dick's defense, a butt-naked-meat-whacking hubby in the background, with me being deaf and hearing all the wrong shit, definitely stacked the odds against me.

Sometime after, just like many of the sex store/gas station drugs, Dick Density was just a high dose of Tadalafil, aka Cialis. So, me taking 100 to 200 milligrams of a medication that was only meant for 20 milligrams was just a waste, and luckily it didn't have side effects that could have been life-threatening. Ironically, Cialis had been working just fine for me in my other sexual situations, so my bootleg boy toy fails were all in my head. In hindsight the boytoy situation was extremely damaging to my ability to use pills for ED help. Not understanding the role anxiety played in making pills ineffective, it created a deep degree of doubt. Taking Viagra/Cialis in these extremely high doses with no success created a negative imprint where I worried every time if the pill would work. Prior to this I was fairly confident, but those days were over. Like I said earlier, if I was confident it would work. If I wasn't it didn't. Simple as that. So if you hit a point where the pills are not working for you, most likely it has nothing to do with the pill. Could be in your head. Pills just open your blood vessels for more blood to flow in and ironically anxiety causes your body to restrict blood flow... and clearly the anxiety is stronger. If you don't believe in your dick, its nothing a pill can do.

Penis Injections

The third route, and I still believe this is an effective route, are injections. I mentioned earlier that my dad was a vet, and he was getting all these prescriptions and giving them to me. One brand I got hold of from him is called Edex, and one is called Caverject. Now, let me be clear: this shit is NOT for everyone!

You need to do these injections right before sex. They come in individual packets with a water base and a powder that you mix in a syringe and inject this mixture into your penis about 10 or 15 minutes before you want an erection. The truth? Even though it works, it is vastly inconvenient.

To most guys, the very idea of injections in your penis is horrifying, but I'll tell you the truth — it sounds worse than what it really is. These brands use a very, very tiny diabetic needle, and if you do it the right way, you don't even feel a thing. If you can get over the whole small needle in your dick thing, the erection you get is implant level. It is some SERIOUS wood.

But it also comes with some serious drawbacks. Number one, as I mentioned earlier, is the inconvenience. Unless you have very regimented sex with your partner at home at a time, you know it's coming, finding a way to prick your dick can be tricky. If you're hooking up with someone that you met in the club and go back to their place, you'll have to carry this shit with you. And when you're all hot and heavy with a woman and you know it's time to get it going, now all of a sudden it's "Excuse me a second; I gotta run to the bathroom."

Well, at least that was my line! I would have to stay in that bathroom way too long, which was kind of a mood killer, but when I would come back out, everything would be good to go. For me, it really killed spontaneity. I'm a guy that likes to have an adventurous sex life—things could pop off in the car, or they could pop off in a restroom somewhere, or anywhere else, so it ended up not being for me.

And here's the killer: we may all think we want the hardest cock we can imagine, but with these injections, you have *no control* over the erection you get depending on your dose. You might even have this erection for two to four hours. It may not fucking go down at all and you got to go to the hospital. The medical name for this actual fucking nightmare is *priapism*.

So when you hear those commercials that talk about ED meds that say, "If you experience an erection for four to six hours, please contact your doctor," they're not fucking around. This stuff is the real thing. I used to hear that and say, "Four to six-hour erection? What the fuck? Who's gonna get that?" But with injections, you can have sex, have an orgasm, have sex again and have an orgasm again, take a nap, wake back up—and still have an erection.

Note that having an erection for too long can cause scarring and damage the blood vessels. I'm sure you don't want to permanently damage your dick. One of the only ways to bring down one of these extended erections is to take multiple Sudafed at once—which ain't good for you at all. I've done that. You might do a shit ton of jumping jacks to make blood flow to other places in your body. I've tried this, too. But if nothing works and you have to go to the hospital, they take a large catheter and put it inside your penis to drain the blood out manually. Yes, this sounds like some medieval Viking shit, but in desperation, I once speared my own junk and bled myself.

Yeah, I'm a gangster, but please don't do what I did.

The Hard Ride Home!

So as you know, my ED hit a point after my shitty story where I couldn't maintain a natural erection to save my life. My dick was a perpetual slinky. (If you're too young to know what a slinky is, Google it…you'll understand my pain.) The part that hit the hardest (pun intended) was my woman hiring a guy to fuck her on my watch. (Well, his huge dick definitely was a close second). Living my life as a sort of sex symbol with all the women after me hit my confidence hard and had me in the gutter of low self-esteem.

So of course, when I randomly got a call from a woman seeking to hire me for sex, I was instantly interested. She was an African woman who owned a nail salon in nearby Pennsylvania and was recently divorced. She said she traveled to New York for fun on the weekends and wanted an arrangement for her sexual needs!

Now, in all my years as a stripper, sex work had not been my thing. My dick, from my teenage years through my prime, has always been a bougie bastard—wanting only the caviar of crotches—"Please pass the Grey Poupon" shit. Plus, once my ED kicked in, that just took it to another level of complication, and my couple of attempts at sex work were mostly all failures.

Now you're probably saying to yourself, "How in the world is this dude going to sell dick, and he got ED?" That is a valid question. I was currently at the rock bottom of my dick function. But in comes dick injections to save the day. When I say these things work, I truly believe you could maintain an erection while set on fire with this stuff. So it's all good.

Also, a big plus in the scenario is I got her to send me a picture, and she was fine as hell. Not Grey Poupon, but definitely Golden's Spicy Brown mustard. So, we arrange a tentative schedule and start to negotiate a price. Now, this was supposed to get me on a high of confidence as a sexy woman buying your dick is the ultimate ego stroke, but my high-end luxury dick feeling immediately took a blow when she started side street flea market style haggling with me on the pay.

And to make matters worse, haggling just hits different in a strong African accent. Selling my dick started to feel like I was buying a fake Rolex out of a suitcase on Canal Street. So, my starting point was a convenient high-end hotel in downtown NYC plus $500 an hour per session. I settled with a 2-hour drive to Pennsylvania, a motel, $150 for the night, and I covered my own gas and tolls. Safe to say I bought the fake Rolex. But honestly, I didn't care. This wasn't about the money or accommodations.

Like I said, my woman went out and bought dick, and somehow, someone buying mine, even off the clearance rack, made me feel better about myself, and that's what I needed. So we started our arrangement, and I began to see her every couple of weeks.

Now, this was a 40-year-old mother of 2 who had just gotten out of a 20-year marriage. She told me her husband was her first and only sexual partner, and whether this was true or not, I could see there was an apparent sexual naivety to her. I thought that would have been a plus for me, as an inexperienced woman should be overwhelmed by my well-traveled, skilled hoe-ness. But the immaturity just made each sex session a mood-killing game of 20 questions.

All through sex, in a strong African accent, I heard, "Why you do that?" "Why that feel good?" "Why you learn that?" "Do that again." "Don't do that again." "Wait, okay... You can do that again, but tell me before you do that again." It was, by far, some of the most awkward sex talk I've ever had! Thank God for those injections, because there's no way I could have kept an erection without them. In spite of the awkward moments, the mission was accomplished. Those injections were a game changer, and each time was a couple of hours of magical dick slinging!

So, on about the fourth time seeing her, she decided to give me the talk. It went, "You clean?" "I hate condoms." "I want to feel you." "I'm clean." "No condom tonight." Now I knew this woman was inexperienced and caught up in the moment, not to mention about 3 glasses of wine in, so it's my job to be the clear thinker in the situation and make the right decision for us, so I did what any responsible adult male would do. "WELP, she seems clean to me; RAW DOG it is!"

Now, she was definitely on to something, because this was, by far, our best sex thus far. No condom sent her satisfaction through the roof, as she was going crazy. I'm looking down at her, shaking and shivering in pleasure, all the while thinking to myself, *Time to renegotiate my contract; raw dick is at least a $50 raise."*

As her eyes rolled to the back of her head while she climaxed powerfully, her whole body trembling, leaving her in a struggle to gain some composure. My confidence and self-esteem jolted like a surge of electricity; I felt on top of the world. As the moment dissipated, she reached and grabbed me by the back of my neck and pulled me somewhat forcefully face to face with her and, in that strong African accent, she said to me, "DO YOU HAVE AIDS?"

"OMG, what if U have AIDS? I'm a MOTHER! Who's going to take care of my kids? BE HONEST! Do you have AIDS?" She asked these questions in an out-of-the-blue frantic interrogation.

"What the fuck?" At first, I thought she was playing as it was so off the wall that she couldn't be serious, but she certainly was. She was having a full-on dirty dick meltdown at my expense.

I sincerely tried to calm her down and assured her I had a clean bill of health, but she just went on and on about her eventually dying from sleeping with me. Now, I understand there are always concerns when you decide to have unprotected sex with someone, but maybe, just maybe, it's a conversation for BEFORE we cross that bridge. Mind you, I was having this whole dysfunctional sexual health interrogation with my dick hard as an aluminum bat.

Injections give me a 2 to 4-hour erection. All hell broke loose about 20 minutes in, so I had possibly 3 hours and 40 minutes' worth of boner left. Usually, having an orgasm and Sudafed can speed up the process, but on this day, neither was available as her paranoid episode led her to ask me to leave (I guess she needed to start writing her will), and I left my Sudafed home. It's 3 a.m. in Pennsylvania, so nowhere is open to buy Sudafed, so with no other option, I decided to go home.

So now, I had to drive two hours back home with the Erection of Life—it was practically poking out of my driver's side window. I drove the speed limit the whole way because the idea of getting pulled over for speeding with a massive fucking erection was just something I was not trying to experience. All I could think about was being the unarmed Black man killed during a routine traffic stop because his boner was mistaken for a concealed weapon. Now there are BLM protests all over the U.S. with protesters stuffing hero bread in their pants, chanting "Hands up, dicks up" and "Justice for his Piece."

Luckily, I made it home safely to my Sudafed. She eventually got back to her senses, and we continued to hang out for a couple of months until things fizzled. For the remainder of seeing her, she was infamously known for that moment as one of my good buddies, when we were in social circles, urged me relentlessly to share this tale. "Bro, you got to tell them about 'AIDS CHICK.'"

Well, there you go, Adam. I told this story for you. The moral of the story is that penis injections are extremely unpredictable and uncontrollable, especially when you are dealing with unpredictable women, so use them at your own risk.

Penis Pumps

As a male stripper, I've used penis pumps for my entire career, but not for erections. To use a penis pump, you stick your penis in a cylinder to create a kind of vacuum seal, and it works almost like a bicycle pump. You pump it up, but it's not like pumping air in—it's pulling air out of the cylinder, and the suction pulls the blood into your penis. The problem is that the erection is artificial, so the minute the vacuum seal is broken, the blood is going to start to dissipate right back out of your penis. So the goal is to use the pump to get as much blood into your penis as possible, and then upon taking your penis out of the pump, you want to have a cock ring—something that fits really tight around the base of your penis—and put it on immediately. That will trap and squeeze the blood into your dick, which then maintains your erection. The tighter and the quicker you can put it on, the better and stronger the erection, and you can have sex and function to some degree. Understand this, though—it's pretty lacking from a typical erection. It's probably not going to be fully hard; it's going to be more like a semi-erection, enough to penetrate and perform the act, but a far cry from a strong erection.

Side Note: One benefit they don't publicize about penis pumps is because you are manually pulling blood into your penis, you can temporarily double the girth of your penis. (Yes, I said double.) As a stripper, I used this concept before my performances. The normal suggested time in a penis pump is about 10-15 minutes. I would go 25-30 minutes, which would swell my dick up. Talking about hot dog to hot sausage instantly. Then I would put on my cock ring and walk around the crowd, and chicks would think I was King Kong Dong. Now, nice rep to have, as the swelling would typically last the rest of the night. I even brought plenty of chicks home and served them the hot sausage. But every now and then, things would become quite confusing, because if the chick stayed over to the next morning and reached down for my sausage for some morning sex, to her surprise, I was back to just a regular ol' hot dog—awkward. One girl I dated over a brief period of time couldn't contain it and just blurted out one day, "Your dick is a chameleon. It's different every time."

Just like the injections, the penis pump totally kills spontaneity, staying in the mood, and in the moment. So unless you have a long-term partner that has a full understanding of what's going on and can be patient with it, it's a process.

I'll touch on this in a later chapter, but penis pumps can be really helpful if you do decide to go for an implant. They can help you to maintain penis size, elasticity, and strength—things you'll want to preserve and cultivate.

Testosterone Replacement Therapy

Testosterone replacement, or TRT, can definitely give you a boost. I mentioned that I've taken this in a previous chapter. This is a little bit advanced, but a lot of guys choose this route and, after some trial and error, have success with it, at least for a time. This is not a quick fix, and it's not an easy fix, because getting TRT to the proper levels is a very nuanced thing. You have to work with your doctor, and it can take months and months of figuring out the right dose to get you there. Hormonal balance is COMPLICATED. Just ask your girlfriend about their PMS or their perimenopause experience—it's complex as fuck, and when you mess around with it, you don't know what you're gonna get.

However, the idea of increasing testosterone is to get you to an optimal place to tweak your sex drive, and it can make you feel fantastic if it's done the right way. It can change your mood, alleviate your ED, and make you feel generally stronger and better. Many guys I've talked to think TRT is a win-win.

We have something called "free testosterone." We have a total test number, and then we have a free test number. Free test is responsible for our libido and the higher the better—I got into this a few chapters above, as well. As we get older and/or if we live an unhealthy lifestyle, our testosterone can decrease (smoking a lot of weed and drinking can lower our testosterone level), which can mess with our libido and sexual desire. Some guys feel like, "Hey, look, I'll just jump on some testosterone replacement and raise these levels up, which then will increase my libido," and this is a smart, viable thing to do for some. If your ED is not caused by a true physical issue, this is a corrective measure that can reinvigorate your desire for sex and your ED, and really your whole zest for life.

I am on TRT myself but can't say I've had a full reinvigoration. I do have friends of the same age that have experienced this, and it's an option to consider. I want to be clear that it's not a 100% fix, but it can be for some. For others, it may not do anything. Consider going to the doc to get your testosterone levels checked, and if they tell you that they are lower than men your age and you're a candidate for TRT, it can be a corrective measure to consider.

Lifestyle Changes

What do I mean by lifestyle? At first, I tried to correct my ED issues naturally, changing my daily routine and choosing healthier options in terms of sleep, nutrition, and fitness. The main thing for me was working out. If you don't want to go the route of testosterone replacement and you're young and fit enough, you can spike your own testosterone levels through exercise with heavy weights and sprints. Certain ways of exercising will send a message to your body to spike your testosterone levels, which has similar effects to taking TRT.

Working out is something that I've done for years, and I did see a spike in my testosterone levels from the heavy training, but for me, it did not result in a correction to my ED. In my case, from a psychological standpoint, I was already a little bit too far gone to get back to the place where I would be happy. There was some improvement, but I never felt totally comfortable and confident about it and continued to have to use other methods.

CHAPTER SEVEN

Learning to Be a Great Lover
(But Not For Overcompensation)

So now you know some shit about me. Since I've spilled my guts out all over the pages of this book, I can tell you that one other thing I've learned to love the shit out of is pleasing my girl like it's *my fucking job*. Not because I don't want her to know that my dick isn't up to snuff (cuz remember, my implant has changed all that), but because what is a bigger turn-on than a turned-on woman? Literally fucking nothing.

Did you know that 80 percent of women don't have orgasms when they sleep with men? That's right, buddy. Chicks call this "the orgasm gap" because more than 95 percent of heterosexual dudes DO orgasm when they have sex. That is a GAP. And only 18.4 percent of women orgasm from vaginal sex alone (that'll be a key point later in this chapter). And did you know that 59 percent of women *fake* orgasms?! Why do *you* think they do this? Because they want to make you feel like you're getting them off. Like you're the big man. Like your masculinity is unstoppable. Women say they fake it because they want their man to feel good and confident, and sometimes just because they're bored and want to get it over with. That is fucking SAD!

(More orgasm stats here: https://pleasurebetter.com/orgasm-statistics/)

Now, there are some good guides online about how to do the mechanics of getting a woman off, so I'm not gonna focus too much on that here. All I'll say, in case it's not clear to you from your Reddit deep dives, is this: IT'S ALL ABOUT THE CLIT. I said above that most women don't orgasm from vaginal sex, and that's because the clitoris is where their nerve endings are, not inside the vagina. The clitoris is a pretty fucking amazing human organ that you should be in awe of. Not only does this thing have 8,000 nerve endings (a lot more than your penis), but its SOLE PURPOSE IS PLEASURE. That's right, my guy. Your dick is multipurpose—it's the pee thing, the pleasure thing, and the making babies thing. But the clitoris, as just one component of a woman's vulva (the outside of the vagina that you can see), is just there to make a lady feel good.

But—and this is key—you usually can't reach the clit just when you fuck 'em.

That's why you can stick your dick in a chick as much as you want and give them a good and hearty fucking, but they still may not get off. The rarest of rare women will cum just from being fucked, because you've got her at some angle where her clit is getting the attention it needs. But mostly, you're gonna need to use your hand or mouth or a toy to get her to cum—and hopefully scream with pleasure. And remember, as the famous book says, *"She Comes First"*— that means you've got to think about how you're going to get her off with your hand or your mouth or her favorite vibrator before you fuck her or while you're fucking her—*before you cum*. This is especially key if you're experiencing premature ejaculation, another common male sexual dysfunction, more common for younger guys.

132

But here's something that's really important to understand. Even if we know that pleasuring the clit is almost universally the thing most women want and need, we gotta learn *what our individual partners want*. I've done pretty extensive personal research on this (wink) and talked to sexologists and sex therapists about it. The most important thing to know is that ALL WOMEN ARE DIFFERENT. It's a "different strokes for different folks" situation here—just because one girl likes her clit stroked hard and fast on the left side doesn't mean the next one you bang is going to want the same thing. You have to ASK. You can ask while you're out to dinner, or when you're sexting, or you can ask as you're on your way downtown. It's okay to say it very directly: "How do you want me to touch you?" Or to start touching them gently, and then ask, "Does it feel good like this?" Most women will tell you exactly how to do it. Then you can ask, "Is this right?" as you learn the rhythms of their body. This goes for one-night stands and sex with your wife of 10 or 20 years. It's never too late to learn how to give your chick the gift of orgasms.

In the next chapter, I talk about the importance of vulnerability and how so much of your sexual-confidence hinges on good communication. Well, communication about pleasure—specifically *her pleasure*—is a huge part of your mental health equation. And what did you learn so far? That your mental health is probably the real reason your dick is failing you. Having confidence about your sexual abilities is probably the number one way to make sure your dick works when it's time to fuck.

So, getting great at getting her off has a selfish fucking side bonus!

CHAPTER EIGHT

Relationship Communication: Talking to
Your Girl About Your Dick Early and Often

So now you know why it's so important to learn how to pleasure your partner, whether you're doing casual hookups or are in bed with a long-term lover. To review—it's not just because you're a generous, sensitive dude that you need to know how to work a clit—it's because getting her needs met gets *your needs met.* And the confidence that gives you can immensely fucking help with erectile dysfunction.

One thing I've experienced again and again and have heard countless stories about is that it can be even more difficult to keep an erection with women that we really care about. When the stakes are higher and the feelings are deeper, we're more invested, and that means our dicks may falter, especially if we've ever had an issue with ED in the past. We really want to impress a woman we care about or see a future with—and specifically, we want to impress them with our hard, dependable cocks. That's what was going on with the woman I wrote about a few chapters ago! I really loved that lady, and that made my dick even more likely to disappoint me—and both of us. Our bodies feel our feelings, and our heart isn't just on our sleeve—it's in our cocks. When we're trying so hard to project virility in these moments, because we think our masculinity is all about hard-as-freezer-meat cocks—it can be damn difficult to stay hard, because our feelings are soft and loving. How do we overcome this if we're sexing women we love and not just chicks we met at the club?

ED can make us feel fucking terrible about ourselves. We might feel guilty that we can no longer perform for our partners, which is one of the crucial ways we feel good about ourselves in relationships. As I've mentioned, a man's sexual performance can make him feel powerful and validated. When these feelings aren't affirmed by our partner, it can feel like a fucking void inside us. We're not going to get that affirmation if we're keeping our creeping or existing ED as a dark secret. If that void starts to form, it can have a domino effect, and if we still can't talk about it—our relationship may not survive. And if it does survive, it'll be a shitty, unfulfilling relationship for both of us.

ED also causes friction in relationships that shows up in other ways that are not obvious. If we have had ED before and we're with a woman for the first time, we might worry that it's going to rear its (shrunken) head again. If we really like a woman, we might be even more worried! Taking Viagra or Cialis can give us confidence the first few times that we're having sex, but it's not ideal to keep taking those drugs every time just for the sake of confidence, and after a while, they might not work as well.

How to Have the Talk

Now, what we need to do is have that conversation with our girl EARLY. If you had an STI, you'd tell a woman you were about to fuck, right? "I got tested, and I am on antibiotics for (*insert your infection here*), but you'll be okay because I'ma put on this condom." Side note: if you're not the kind of person who'd tell them, you're an actual piece of shit.

It's the same thing for ED. You can't hide it from someone you're dating that you'll be sleeping with in an ongoing way, so don't even try. This is also the case if you've been with the same chick for a decade. If you're starting to experience ED, you should tell them about it. There is NO SHAME in this, as I keep telling you. It's not going to make you weaker, or your relationship weaker—it's only going to strengthen your bond. The question is—how do you do it?

If you don't tell your partner about your ED, those feelings of failure, rejection, shame, and anxiety could begin to spiral out of control and then WAY out of control. At some point, we might realize that we're just not fucking our partner anymore. First it dwindles to once a week, then once a month, then once every six months, and suddenly a year has passed and you haven't fucked your girl. I don't ever want you to get to this place, no matter what you eventually decide to do about your ED—whether you follow my lead and get an implant or use other methods. If you want your relationship to survive and thrive, or if you want a woman you think you might fall for to stick around, this is how you can have the ED talk.

First of all, don't do it in bed, or in or around sexy times. Choose a time where you're both relaxed, not rushing out anywhere, and maybe both sitting at the kitchen table or far from the bedroom. You probably won't want to have this convo when you're out to dinner or in public. Privacy is key, so if you have kids, do it when they're out or asleep and you know they won't bother you for a while.

136

Start by saying, "I want to talk to you about this, but it's hard for me, so please give me some space to be vulnerable, okay?" If your woman is decent, she'll lap that up and open her whole heart to you right then. Tell her you love her, and you value the relationship above all else. Tell her you're still wildly attracted to her. Then explain that things have started to change for you and you're not getting or staying hard like you used to (depending on exactly where you are and what your issue is when you have this talk). Tell her if you've decided to start taking Viagra or Cialis, and that she might see packages around the house. Tell her if you've started thinking about using a penis pump. You may want to add in some facts about how common ED is—and if you're in your late thirties or older, how insanely common it is for people your age. Throw in a recent statistic from this book for good measure.

Now, this may end up being the beginning of a longer conversation, or maybe you'll just talk about it one time, and you'll both feel good about working on your sex life together, now that she knows what you're dealing with. Be open to doing couples therapy or seeing a sexologist or sex coach for direction and tips that are more specific to your own unique situation. Most relationships that have already started to erode *can be fixed*, especially if there is love there and there was real attraction from the start. Be patient, and know it may take a while to get your groove back together.

Fellas, I know this may be uncomfortable, and the idea of doing this may make you cringe, but if you love your woman, do it for her. Telling your woman what's going on avoids a ton of confusion, and I'm sure she will be relieved to understand it's not her and be very receptive to helping with finding a way to get through it together.

The erosion of our sex lives can lead to resentment, insecurity, a lack of feeling desired by both parties, and a bunch of other very depressing shit. When we feel like our sexuality is slipping away, the pressure can create a passive wedge that slowly and agonizingly destroys the relationship. Disagreements might fester and linger. An argument that would normally last twenty-four to forty-eight hours could turn into a week, then two weeks, then three weeks…you get the picture?

As men, it is usually our job to fix these little spats. To reach for our partners in a healing, loving way. This can result in a moment of intimacy—make-up sex is hot! But ED that we haven't talked about can subconsciously prevent us from making that move. This is yet another reason to have that talk as soon as you're aware of your issue.

Being a male stripper, I cannot tell you the number of women I come across who are in sexless marriages. I know this happens for various reasons, but I also know that a lot of this acceptance of sex ending in the relationship is a byproduct of diminishing sexual performance and chemistry with their husbands, which wasn't proactively addressed and ultimately results in both giving up on sex completely.

Avoiding the Void

If you don't try to repair this space, both partners are left to fill their voids outside of the relationship. It becomes the focus of many partners to supplement that need for intimacy and fulfillment.

Like I mentioned earlier, men with ED in our diminished state—we're more likely to cheat. I know that sounds confusing, as one would question: if you can't perform at home, why would you go out and seek it elsewhere to fail? Cheating in this way is another attempt to avoid the pressure of the sexual decline. There is pretty universal devastation among women who learn that their spouse with performance issues, who's given up on sex with her, is now engaging elsewhere.

Because the guy was too embarrassed to talk about it in the first place, she's gonna assume he lost attraction or desire for her. This creates all kinds of insecurity, shame, and self-esteem issues for the woman. In most cases, they're just completely wrong and making assumptions because they were never given the truth in the first place.

We are not the only ones in the relationship aging or dealing with confidence issues, etc. As I touched on earlier about the "beauty myth," women deal with their own struggles with how the world gives them standards to live up to. It's extremely important for your woman to feel desired and lusted for by you. The loss of that belief can cause all types of issues for her that can be damaging to her self-esteem and mental health. So if you suddenly become avoidant of sex, or there's a drop-off in your initiating/aggression to be sexual with her, she can easily feel unwanted or rejected by you, and now you both are going through it. At the start of a relationship, you tend to perform at a higher rate sexually. This "honeymoon phase" is when most of our connection, confidence, and security is created. You set a standard for yourself as a lover that you may take for granted. But as our performance deteriorates, pressure can grow. A man wants to please his woman. He wants to maintain a certain degree of performance, and the truth is, we would rather not do it than fail at it.

In cheating situations, when a dude finds a random chick or escort or whatever his means of cheating is, there's no pressure. Who cares about your performance during a one-night thing? There's a much lower level of satisfaction you're required to meet. There's a much lower standard, so you feel more comfortable than you do in your actual relationship. A lot of this infidelity could probably be avoided on both sides if a man steps up and has that conversation with his partner early, so they can work on it together.

In short, HAVE THAT TALK. It's never too late, and it can never be too early. It might just save your relationship and your sex life.

CHAPTER NINE

Aging is Normal: Learning to Love Your Older, Wiser Dick

This book is for guys of all ages, but I know my older brothers are probably the ones who will pick it up first. I'm over fifty, coming at you with my years of wisdom, and a lot of my friends are in my age group, recently divorced, with kids, and just getting back out there to date, only to realize that their dick isn't what it was in their twenties.

Now, this change happens over time, and if they were paying closer attention, they might have realized that shit was shifting when they were in their mid-to-late thirties, but they were so busy being dads and husbands and working that it just kinda slipped by them. Suddenly they're waking up alone in their bachelor pad and swiping through Hinge only to meet up with a woman and find out their dick doesn't work! Or maybe their kids went away to college, and they want to rekindle the sexual spark with their wife, only to find that they can't get it up. It can be a shock to the system, but it's far from the end of anyone's sex life.

Ageism Is Bullshit

Now, life for men is difficult as it is, and the path we take to developing a good solid life we can be proud of is usually a long and difficult one. The years put in to acquire knowledge, wisdom, and patience. The house, car, nice bank account, and the true flexibility to enjoy life arrive for most later in life. Now, I can truly sit back and enjoy the fruits of my labor. Thank you, universe... it all worked out for me... except, why did you choose now for my dick to start acting up? I mean... could the timing be more shitty?

So now I have to get up every day with life appearing to be perfect, not a care in the world because I paid my dues, worked hard, and secured my future. But Father Time is one cruel bastard because this ageism thing is usually a trade-off: I reached the mountaintop, but it was no working dicks allowed. This gets into the shame that I've been talking about in a lot of different chapters in this book. A lot of people have shame about aging because our fucking society makes us think that old people don't matter, and only young people's lives are interesting and worth paying attention to. The quality of your sex life is not a priority as you age. And one of an older man's biggest secrets is the immense shame he may feel about his dick.

So let's get proactive, so when you reach your destination of "I'm officially living good, and my hard work paid off," you can get hard and enjoy life to the absolute fullest. Here are a few tips to pay attention to on this journey.

The Importance of Morning Wood

Your penis is a muscle: that's why men get spontaneous erections all night long. When a man goes to sleep, he can have three to seven erections throughout the night, lasting twenty to thirty minutes at a time. This is a sign of good health that has zero to do with being horny—it ain't mysterious at all.

Since the penis is a muscle, our younger body automatically says, "Hey look, we need to exercise this thing." So your body goes through its own maintenance schedule of giving you an erection, which moves your blood, wrestles, and stretches the skin, blood vessels, and the tip —this is how your dick maintains its length, fullness, and rigidity. If you're not getting these erections, just like when you don't go to the gym, your dick eventually starts to atrophy and shrink and gets smaller just because it's not being used.

Now guess what happens as we age? Exactly that. After our twenties, our nighttime erections happen much less often. So not only are we more prone to erectile dysfunction, our dick may be shrinking!

So if you noticed you stopped getting morning erections, that is a clear sign you're on the decline and your dick is telling you, "Hey, look, you need to correct your ED before you get to a point where you can't get an erection." Once you hit that point where your penis no longer gets hard, and you let it stay limp for long periods of time, your blood vessels are going to shrink, your skin is going to shrink, and your capacity for your penis to get fully erect is going to shrink.

So this is me telling you that you need to get started on prepping your dick in your thirties and early forties. One way to do some age-appropriate prevention? Use your dick whenever you can! Masturbating regularly can help to keep your dick muscle in better shape, just like lifting at the gym. If you can still get an erection, this is a great way to prime the pump. You can do this even when you're not horny, in the shower once a day, or some other time that works for you.

There are a lot of anti-science conspiracy theories that masturbation is bad for you—the movement is called "no fap," and I'm here to call complete bullshit on it. If you see one of these threads in a forum, walk on by. Masturbation is GOOD FOR YOU.

Shrinkage Doesn't Just Happen in the Pool

What if you're reading this book because your situation is already pretty far gone and you're having trouble getting erections at all? There are solutions for you, too. I know aging men who eventually got implants but lost their erections completely and went two years, three years, four years without getting one. By the time they get the implant, their dick is atrophied and smaller. It's a fucking nightmare for these guys.

Let's say before, when their penis was working, normally it was six inches long, and now, since it hasn't been erect for five years, the skin and the muscle are atrophied. So when they get an implant, the biggest implant they can get is only four and a half inches because their penis no longer can stretch and fill up to its full ability.

But there's something that guys in this situation can do: a penis pump! If you're suffering from ED, considering an implant or not, this is one way to start training your dick again if you can't get an erection naturally. Use that penis pump for twenty minutes a day, and it will start to re-stretch your dick. It will stretch the skin and artificially pull blood into your penis and hold it there as long as it's in the pump cylinder. This will begin to re-stretch the erection.

When I have friends who are waiting for approval for the implants, I tell them, "Bro, go out, buy a pump immediately."

144

Even urologists usually give this advice. So by the time you get the implant, you'll be able to hopefully get back to your normal size or close.

An implant always brings happiness. "Hey, I can use it again." "I can have sex again." But you still run into that scenario of it's not what I expected or I'm not the person I'm used to being if you lost size from prolonged inactivity. I don't know anybody that would be happy with losing some size off their dick. Once again, this is me telling you not to let this fester and don't let your dick shrink!

Remember, I wrote this book to help you be proactive. Don't wait. It is an epidemic. I cannot get on the phone with anyone over thirty-three who is not experiencing some kind of erectile dysfunction. There are guys in their late twenties already doing Viagra or Cialis or venturing into any gas station or bodega buying penile erection enhancement over-the-counter drugs. So start thinking about the health of your dick early. If you're young, or if you're getting on in years, remember that it's never too late to take care of your dick—because a healthy functioning dick will definitely take care of you.

CHAPTER TEN

How My Implant Saved My Life
(But Your Solution May Be Different)

The Dick Avengers

So here we are, at my favorite part of the story. The part where I get to talk joyously about my implant and all things associated with it. I'm so very excited! (Happy dance takes place). See, the powerful way a penis implant changes your life is very hard to describe to someone. The best way I can sum it up is by using a movie analogy, and my Marvel fans will definitely get where I'm coming from; all others, just try to follow along.

In *Marvel's Avengers: Infinity War*, the God of Thunder, Thor—who for the longest time had been considered the most powerful Avenger in the Marvel Universe—has been through some serious battles, so he is clearly not in his most powerful form. Most importantly, the main source of his power, his magical hammer given to him by his father to channel his power, has been destroyed in a previous battle by a treacherous female villain.

Everyone who follows *Marvel* knows that Thor without his hammer is a shell of his power capabilities. Early in this movie, Thor encounters Thanos, an all-powerful supervillain who kills Thor's loved ones and leaves him floating in space to die. Luckily, Thor is rescued and vows revenge, but in order to defeat Thanos, he needs not only a new hammer, but a more powerful one.

So, Thor sets out to travel to a planet where the most powerful weapons are created. He subjects himself to near death by channeling the energy of a star through his body to create the heat needed to forge his new hammer. The weapon is made, and as Thor is holding onto the last breaths of his life, the weapon is placed in his hand, and a powerful surge of energy shoots through his body. Not only is the Mighty Thor back alive and strong, but he is by far the most powerful version of himself because he wields the most powerful weapon any man has held to channel his power through. He now has the STORMBREAKER—half hammer and half axe, and nothing to be messed with. It's a weapon more than capable of killing Thanos, the villain who left him for dead.

To clarify the comparison: I was Thor, and at some point, my hammer (dick) was destroyed by a treacherous female villain (my ex-girlfriend). In this weak state, Thanos showed up(just life and the pressures we face as men starting over, meeting women, or maintaining current relationships while dealing with ED) and left me for dead(depressed with anxiety about my ED, making me feel insecure and unwanted).

But like Thor, I wanted revenge and refused to give up and let Thanos win, so I traveled to the planet of weapons(the implant doctor), channeled the power of a star (did whatever was needed financially and mentally for the surgery to happen), then walked out, similar to Thor, with the most powerful weapon: the Stormbreaker (my implanted dick is a weapon that makes me the most powerful version of myself—period!). I know the Avenger analogy is probably entertaining, especially for the Marvel fans reading, but I can't be more serious when I say this shit is life -changing. Just imagine the best erection you have ever had, but make it better, and it only goes down if you want it to. It's really unfair. I tap out EVERY woman I have sex with effortlessly. Never at any point in my life, with my natural penis, could I come close to this sexual potency. Wouldn't you want this unbelievable sexual ability? The power to produce an erection you would imagine belongs to a superhero. I certainly think so, and through this book, I'm trying to create a movement—a team to fight against the struggles of men all over by correcting your ED, getting your own Stormbreaker, and defeating the Thanos of your life!

Remember, Thanos is inevitable… so if you want to beat him, you can join me and be a Dick Avenger in your own little multiverse.

All our stories may be different, but we have the same goal: to defeat Thanos by being our most powerful selves. So, whether Iron Man, The Incredible Hulk, or Captain America is your character of choice, I urge you to join the team, and we'll defeat Thanos together.

The Infinity War is over, and it's the ENDGAME now. So, in the great words of Captain America, "AVENGERS… ASSEMBLE!" Now we all scream at the top of our lungs and run into battle, aka fix our dicks!

Okay, okay… I couldn't resist my Marvel movie sales pitch, but here's the process to really get it done if you want to correct your ED once and for all.

So, if you've read this far, you understand that I'm kind of a penis implant evangelist—mainly because it entirely changed my life for the better, as have countless men I've counseled about implants, and I've watched them change their lives too (my dad was first on that list). Even with that said, it should be your last resort because it's the type of operation that once you do it, there is no turning back.

As we know, there are lots of psychological approaches, medical options, and over-the-counter remedies for ED, but in my experience, they tend not to work at all or work for a short time before they no longer do. That's why I haven't gone into much detail about these remedies in this book—because, in my experience, they're only a temporary and often problematic fix. Occasionally, I talk to a dude who loves his Viagra and has been loving it for a decade with no problems—so if that's you, God bless.

That's not the vast majority of men. If you are the guy who has given up on these options and find yourself avoiding sex and intimacy, this is for you.

The one thing you'll probably experience if you decide to get an implant is that if you go straight to your doctor and say, "Doc, please take my money and give me an implant," you'll be turned away the first time. This is par for the course—don't give up!

Before going to the doctor, you must start with a plan at home. Most doctors are going to tell you no because it's unethical to just give someone an implant, especially if you are under 65 years old. For how amazing this surgery works, it has primarily only been offered to older men after prostate surgery, so someone my age at the time—47—is not the usual candidate.

If you haven't had a prostate procedure, you need to show a history of trying to remedy it yourself and that you tried every option available. This is the main reason why penis implants are so uncommon.

Insurance companies don't want to foot the bill, so they want to see that you tried every avenue before they approve it. A history of Viagra/Cialis, then injections like Caverject or Edex, are usually needed as a minimum to start the consideration. So, if you want your insurance to consider you as a candidate, get to your doctor and start receiving prescriptions for ED meds. After receiving these meds, if they work…great! But if not, follow up with your doctor and make sure he knows you're unhappy with the results.

Once you exhaust pills and injections (say pills don't work and injections cause painful erections, if any), then you are a candidate to be approved. Without that history, it's a no-go.

Now, in my case, I paid out of pocket, so I didn't have to go through the insurance song and dance. However, even my first time going to the doctor for a consultation to inquire about it, I was told no and left there with a prescription for Cialis. Now this is not a fact, but I think the reason I was initially turned down and prescribed Cialis is that the doctor was covering his own ass.

He probably needed some sort of medical history of him trying to treat my ED by another means as opposed to just immediately giving me the implant. But at this point, I was determined to get the surgery, so I returned after a few months and got the process going.

At the time, the cost was $32,000, which was really high for the procedure, as most out -of -pocket costs were $16,000 to $20,000. But I wanted to go to the best doctor available. (If you are already balking at the price, just think: $16,000–$32,000 is a decent used car these days. Ask yourself—do you want a Camry in the garage or a Porsche in your pants?)

We are talking about my dick, so this is not the time to bargain hunt, so I went with the best doctor available. For the $32,000, I paid $12,000 cash and financed the other $20,000. Most offices have some sort of finance company they work with to pay for surgery over time (yes, I have a Dick Note and I'm still making payments).

It is extremely important to choose a high-volume surgeon—a guy who has done hundreds of surgeries. The more experience, the better—it's important to make sure your dick is in the right hands (says the male stripper who's been dick -groped by strangers for two decades). Do as I say, not as I do!

But seriously, please find the best doctor possible if you can. My doctor did something really cool: he gave me a booklet of all previous patients who volunteered to speak to people considering the surgery. It had around 500 names and numbers broken up by age and ethnicity.

I really wanted to talk to someone, so I reached out to four people, and the conversations confirmed that I was making the right decision.

These four men, all between 70 and 85 years old, responded like they were reading from a script. Unanimously, they proclaimed it was the best decision they ever made, that I was going to love it, and they wished they had done it sooner… and when I told them I was 47, they all went crazy. One specifically said, "Good gravy on the table! If I had this thing at your age, all hell would have broke loose." All of these guys had been implanted for between 15 and 20 years with no issues. After those calls, it was a done motherfucking deal.

151

Once I was scheduled to have the procedure, it started with a couple of tests. One test is called a Doppler test. It's basically an MRI of your penis, so the doctor can see if you have any complications, blood flow issues, or if you have something called a venous leak, which means blood is leaking out of your penis when you get an erection. This test also checks whether you have scar tissue, trauma, or pain. Finding something on this test is actually a good thing for people with insurance, as it provides a justified reason to get the surgery.

Scar tissue was something I thought might have been an issue for me because I was a male performer. I mentioned earlier that I would often use a penis pump and tie off my penis to maintain an erection while at work. I worried that this could have caused damage, but again, I didn't have any physical issues. My issues were truly all psychological.

Take note: when your ED is psychological, your doctor may not want to give you an implant, but in severe cases, they can get it approved. Mine was a severe case because I had been battling it for years.

Once they conduct the MRI, they also test you with one of the injectables to create an erection so the doctor can take a measurement. Based on this erection, he will know what size implants you will need. Implants are typically measured in centimeters, and a good doctor will be able to size you correctly based on the measurements and MRI scan.

They may also give you a test called a cystoscopy (especially if you're older) to make sure your urination flow is normal. This is a test they generally give if you're already having some kind of incontinence or not urinating fully. I was able to bypass that test because of my age. If you're good to go after all these tests, they will green -light your surgery. I was able to schedule mine within two to three weeks of my consultation.

The Surgical Procedure

First and foremost, there are different kinds of implant devices. You should only consider a 3-piece device, and the brands are AMS and Coloplast. If a doctor offers you anything other than a 3-piece device, refuse. The 3-piece devices are the most advanced and really look and operate like your natural penis. So, in my opinion, it's the best way to go. The surgery itself is extremely simple and, in most cases, is completed in under an hour.

Basically, it involves placing inflatable cylinders in the penis shaft. The inflatable cylinders connect to a reservoir filled with saline solution that is placed by your bladder, and a pump is hidden in the scrotum. When you press on the pump, the saline solution travels to the device and inflates it, giving you an erection.

Penises become erect in three locations. In the shaft of the penis, there are two columns, like straws, called the corpus cavernosum. They run the length of your penis from the tip to deep in your scrotum on either side of your urethra and contain vessels that fill with blood to help make an erection. The other part of the penis that becomes erect is the spongy tissue that runs through the shaft of the penis, which engorges, giving it form and girth. The third part of the erection is the tip. All three areas become erect in their own way and each from a different kind of blood flow. When you get an implant, the doctor is only working with the two columns (i.e., corpus cavernosum), which are solely responsible for length and rigidity. The other parts will still receive their own blood flow from sexual excitement and engorge on their own.

Depending on the doctor, they might make a very small incision in the testicles, along the center crease, to access the bottom of the two straws (corpus). Then, they'll create a small incision at the bottom of each corpus and use a tool to hollow them out to make space for the cylinders.

Next, the doctor will take the cylinders made from the measurements obtained from the tests they performed before surgery, insert them into each of the corpus, place the reservoir and the pump in position, and suture up the incision.

Another place the doctor can make the incision to implant the device is on the top of the base of the penis. I chose the testicles because my research suggested that this method offers the best healing scenario; it results in a better scar situation, and some doctors believe it allows you to maintain as much length as possible.

On the day of the surgery, it's a normal routine: you're not going to eat the night before, and you're going to get there early. They'll give you a dose of antibiotics because cleanliness is paramount for this surgery, and warding off infections is essential. It goes without saying that you want to use a very experienced doctor who has a technique that ensures the most sanitized scenario because an infection can be catastrophic, requiring the removal of the implant and months of healing before you can have a new one.

Post-surgery Recovery

After my surgery, I woke up with some discomfort. My penis was wrapped up like a mummy and pointed straight up. Different doctors use different healing techniques. Some will tell you to stay wrapped up for several weeks and come back to teach you how to use the device. I used a doctor in New York City who is very aggressive with his process. He wraps you up, sends you home with some painkillers, and instructs you to lie on your back for the first forty-eight to seventy-two hours—stay down, do very little, and ensure you slow it all the way down.

Obviously, you have an incision in your testicles, and getting up and moving around can increase blood flow, making it harder to reach the surgical device. You're also sent home with a catheter in your urethra, which means, depending on your doctor, twenty-four to seventy-two hours of emptying the bag.

Don't get me wrong: they want you on your back as much as possible. But once you take the catheter out, you can get up to use the bathroom. In my case, I just had a bottle that I could use in bed or wherever I wouldn't necessarily have to get up and walk to the bathroom.

To expand a little on how the device works: I already explained that two cylinders are placed on either side of the corpus cavernosum. During the procedure, they attach the cylinders to two things. One cylinder is attached to a pump that is placed in your testicles and used to inflate and deflate your implant. The pump is connected to a reservoir that will be filled with fluid—enough fluid to fill the implant to capacity.

Our bodies have some empty space next to our bladder, so the doctor puts the reservoir next to the bladder. The reservoir is where the fluid will rest until you're ready to use it. It's inside you. You don't feel it or see it—there's no indication it's there at all. Now, the pump is about an inch long and there's a little ball on the end, which is about the size of one of your testes. It gives you the feeling that you have three nuts, but it is very inconspicuous. Women you sleep with will see and feel no difference. It is placed toward the back of your scrotum, and to inflate your penis, you just squeeze the little ball about 15 to 40 times to achieve your erection.

To deflate, there's a button also located on the pump you push while holding the shaft, giving it a squeeze and a push. Then, all the fluid will return to the reservoir.

When I went home for healing, my doctor wanted me to use the implant as soon as possible. So, during my three days of healing, I was instructed to get into the tub with very warm water and inflate and deflate the device three times a day for twenty to thirty minutes. The reason for this is that anytime you have surgery, your body wants to heal and tends to heal with scar tissue. In this scenario, if I just let it heal for long periods of time without inflating and deflating, my penis might heal at its current size. So now, when I inflate and deflate, I can have the length I'm accustomed to.

Also, if I didn't inflate and deflate, my penis could be stuck in that position. This is relatively rare, but it can happen.

My doctor specifically wanted me to use it as soon as possible to ensure I retained as much length as I started with. So, I was inflating and deflating by day three, and I will tell you that was where the pain was. Those first seven days of inflating and deflating were horrifically painful. I'm not going to downplay it, and it makes sense because my body was trying to heal. My penis was healing and developing scar tissue. Using the pump to inflate and deflate tore up the scar tissue. But it's very necessary because you don't want it to heal stiff; you want it to heal supple. You need that to happen to heal properly. So, I'd sit in the tub and relax.

Now, it was painful—not just uncomfortable. Obviously, I could have mitigated it with pain meds, but I'm not big on taking medications. But for those seven days, the pain was worth it. The more you use the pump in the early stages, I was told, the more you will retain your natural size, and that was important to me.

Note: your implant doesn't increase the size of your penis; it makes what you have work at its best capacity. However, some people did not exercise or inflate it enough after surgery, so they ended up losing a half inch or some of their length. Don't be that guy who loses length because you didn't elongate it enough or early enough by using the pump when your doctor told you to. Fun fact: most guys will regain the length over time, but why wait?

After the first seven days of using it, the pain gradually decreases. Most doctors will tell you to resume your sexual activity based on your tolerance for discomfort or pain within two to three weeks.

Now, each doctor will have their own protocol, and I urge you to follow it closely. I can only share mine specifically with the reasoning behind it, but please use it as a reference with your doctor.

Your New Dick

My first experience with my new dick was uncomfortable physically but extremely gratifying mentally. Listen, when I was told I could use it for the first time in two weeks, I did, literally, in two weeks and one minute. Everything was healed; everything was functioning. But there was still definitely some soreness, and I had a slight loss of sensation; so the first time I used it, I did not have my full sensation recovered.

Although I was able to use the implant after two weeks and a minute, I might have been getting as low as 60% of the sensation that I received before having it. But as far as using it in a successful sexual scenario, it was beyond anything I could have imagined. It was amazing. The erection you get is by far the hardest you've ever had in your life, and you are in complete control of it. Any man knows that all erections are not created equal, and this device gives you your personal best every day, every time.

To add to that, it provides pleasure for your partner on a level that is much higher than normal. We all have experienced that moment when you're having sex with your partner, and you're about to cum, and somehow, she feels it and reaches climax too. This happens because when a man is about to climax, our dicks harden up at that moment, providing a greater sensation. With an implant, that extra rigidity you get when you're about to cum is now there with every stroke, every time. It's really unfair.

But more importantly, what it does for you mentally is everything. Most men, our entire lives, battle some form of anxiety when it comes to sex. If you're older, you worry about getting hard or whether you will be good for round two. When you are younger, it's: will I cum too fast, or am I good enough? With this implant and a combination of years of experience, I can say this is truly the first time in my life I've experienced sex completely free of stress and anxiety, and that alone has made sex so much better.

It took me a few months to regain all my sensation, and that's not necessarily the norm because my dad's sensation was exactly the same his first time using it, if not slightly better. If you do lose any sensation, chances are it will return to normal over time and may even be better because a more rigid penis can provide you more pleasure, too.

Self-esteem Takes Time

Now, for me, the self-esteem thing took time. Just like someone who was overweight the majority of their life finally focuses on diet and exercise, loses weight, and looks fantastic, it can still take time to improve that place of insecurity. Their extreme weight loss will eventually improve their self-confidence, but it probably will not skyrocket right away just by looking in the mirror. It takes time to regain self-esteem that has been battered for so long.

Even with my implant, my thought process didn't do a complete 180. It took time to rebuild my confidence. During those first few months, I would still take Cialis every time I had sex because, while my penis was taken care of, my mind was not. I was still in a place of psychogenic trauma. I share this to make it clear that serious mental damage can be done when you struggle for years with ED, and even with an implant, the struggle continued for months before I could truly be free of the years of worry and anxiety.

My dad, however, you couldn't tell him shit. From day one, he was good! The implant is undeniable. If you do it, you're going to be all right. However, if you've gotten here after a long, complicated, rough ride through dark places, there's probably still more work to do on your mental health. There's nothing wrong with therapy!

The truth of the matter is, just having the implant, over time, because of its reliability, will make a huge difference for you. When you don't have to question it and don't have to worry or second-guess whether it's going to work, it creates the space for you to mentally adjust, heal, and get past it a lot sooner. And if you're lucky enough to be like me, you will have the chance to make up for some serious opportunities you missed out on!

VIN-DICK-CATION

As you found out earlier, I achieved a great feat in my journey through life by becoming the first-ever Dickicorn. Far from my finest moment, but if there is a god in charge of sexual moments, he was clearly shining on me. About a year after my implant, I got a random call from the same hot Dominican girls who anointed me the Dickicorn. Gabriella was in town visiting her cousin Ericka, and they wanted to stop by the club to hang out.

Now I was ecstatic about this possibility because they clearly ran into Thor without his hammer during our first encounter, and now I had the STORM-MOTHERFUCKING-BREAKER! They met me at the club, we bar hopped a bit, and after way too many drinks, they actually admitted to me that they still laugh about what happened, and I'm not even known by my actual name. Over the years, I've been referred to simply as Dickhead: "Remember the time with Dickhead?" "Me and Dickhead follow each other on IG," and that led to us hanging out: "Let's give Dickhead a call and hang out."

Now I took this in stride, as I can take a joke with the best of them, It definitely landed much softer knowing I had a never-ending erection in my pants.

That same conversation, without my implant, would have left me with a spontaneous sex change and shriveled my penis to the size of a clit. Nonetheless, I'm good. So, as the dick gods continued to favor me, we ended up back at my place, and Ericka was back to her usual tricks, demanding yet again that I fuck her cousin while she watches.

But this time, there was no screaming like the *Home Alone* kid. Not a drop of fear, worry, or anxiety existed in my being. I just calmly reached down to my balls in a very inconspicuous way, gave my balls about 40 furious pumps, and dropped my jeans. They both gasped at the magnificence of my penis as it stood at attention like a soldier during the national anthem.

Needless to say, I took a page out of Dee and Dug's WWE smackdown sex performance and went Hulk Hogan royal rumble on their vajayjays. Within 45 minutes, not only did they tap out, but they were begging for mercy: "No mas, papi, no mas!" Just call me Sugar Ray Leonard, as I brought the Roberto Duran to the bedroom (if you're too young to understand this, kick rocks). This moment was the sweetest form of vindication imaginable.

I went from the first-ever Dickicorn to Mr. Por Favor No More. Sometimes the world just aligns perfectly, and this was as sweet as it gets!

CONCLUSION

Curing ED is more than just resolving an erection issue. It's a mental health problem that is crippling men all across the world. The effects of it are not just sexual; it creates all types of severe mental and emotional issues for men, aside from the physical aspects.

As men, we're taught to keep these feelings bottled up and not to express them, not to speak about them, and not to truly seek help in a way that is beneficial to us. We kind of just live in this place of despair, struggling through the loss of, for most of us, the most essential part of our being.

A man without sexuality is a shell, and a shell of yourself is nothing we should ever settle for. We should do everything in our power to remedy it by any means necessary. If your efforts are anything short of that, you are doing yourself a disservice.

We strive for success and to be the best we can be in almost every aspect of our lives. Between work, home, finances, athletics, competition, etc., we want to win. We want to be the best. Even if we don't actively try to, we want to. When it comes to your sexuality, it's not a choice. You have to do it.

Don't settle for a life where you are diminished in that essence and in that very crucial part of your being. You have to be in it for self-preservation because it's the only way to ensure that it's intact and stays intact.

The decision to get an implant is not an easy one for most of us. But when you receive the information about it, how it's presented, and the improvements that have been made in science, you will see how it can totally reinvent you, restoring your sexual abilities, confidence, and all the things that were essential to you as a young man that you took for granted.

Once you make the decision and experience it, the only thing you'll question is, "Why didn't I do this a long time ago?" It is a no-brainer. The bottom line is this: as men, we need to bring this to full attention and get it done as frequently as a normal procedure like breast implants.

No one thinks twice about it. Everybody celebrates nice breasts. The world should also celebrate a rock-hard dick, just like I celebrate mine every day. So, I'm trying to open the door. I want to slam the door open, and for my fellas out there struggling with these issues—to run to it. Break the door down.

Let's change this dynamic and bring back our masculinity, our sense of security, confidence, and vitality. Stop hiding in the dark, trying to avoid this problem with one pill at a time. Stop. It's time. Let's do this!

There you have it. My E(D) True Floppywood Story.

I genuinely hope I was able to help someone out there by sharing my life struggles in such an unfiltered way. It was truly my goal to be a voice… hopefully a loud one that normalizes a man's decline in a personable, relatable, entertaining way. For years, this was my huge secret...so much so that it was a secret I hid from myself. It's easier to fool yourself into believing everything is fine than to shamefully struggle with it. Listen, if I could be arrogant for a moment, I was the fucking man! My life résumé said I had it all. I was a winner. But even with that said... without my dick, I never felt more like a loser. Call me shallow, call me a douche, call me anything you want, but when I got implanted and regained my erection, I swear to you... the physical fix was the smallest impact compared to the way it improved my life. It was so much greater—my confidence, my masculinity, my drive, my belief in myself as a worthy partner, and my feeling like a winner again. Why is all this connected to our dicks? I have no idea, but I do know it's time to make it clear that it is and to stop acting like it's not. I hope my story has motivated you to open the refrigerator of life to search and find your freezer meat!

ABOUT THE AUTHOR

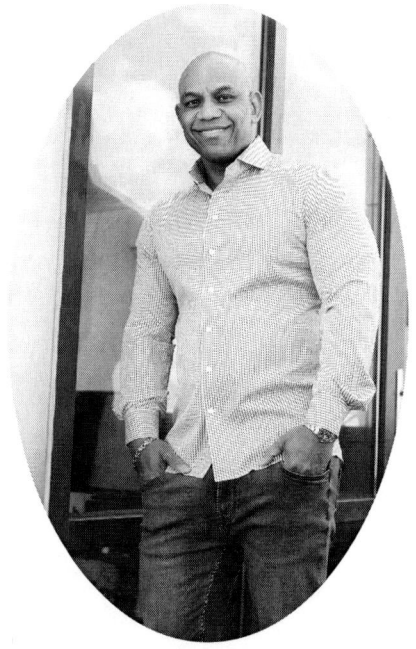

Sharay "Punisher" Hayes

So I understand that this is the part where I'm supposed to drop my resume and qualifications to make myself look good—and you'll learn all those details as you read the book. But first and foremost, I want to say that I see myself as just a guy with what I believe is a powerful message, delivered through very personal stories about my life.

That life includes being a celebrity-level male stripper for 30 years, a reality TV personality, a real estate investor, a business owner, and—most importantly—a womanizing, emotionally traumatized man.

My journey has allowed me to experience the highs and lows of life in a broad way, and it created a perspective that, although our specific details may differ, the core experiences are common and shared by all men. Along the way, I figured out some very important things about masculinity, self-worth, and sexuality as a man—things I believe will resonate with you on a human level.

I'm just here hoping that my wins, losses, and the solutions I've found up to this point in my life might help you—whether it's feeling better about yourself, understanding someone you care about a little more, or avoiding some of the challenges I went through.

I conquered through self-help, and now I'm here to encourage self-help in others.

Thank you sincerely for your time and interest in my life, my opinions, and my message. I hope you enjoy reading it as much as I enjoyed living it.

Made in United States
North Haven, CT
16 April 2026

10102845R00109